T0259496

Toxicology Testing

Guest Editor

MICHAEL G. BISSELL, MD, PhD, MPH

CLINICS IN LABORATORY MEDICINE

www.labmed.theclinics.com

September 2012 • Volume 32 • Number 3

SAUNDERS an imprint of ELSEVIER, Inc.

W.B. SAUNDERS COMPANY
A Division of Elsevier Inc.

1600 John F. Kennedy Boulevard • Suite 1800 • Philadelphia, Pennsylvania 19103-2899

http://www.theclinics.com

CLINICS IN LABORATORY MEDICINE Volume 32, Number 3
Septemebr 2012 ISSN 0272-2712, ISBN-13: 978-1-4557-4960-7

Editor: Teia Stone

Reprints. For copies of 100 or more, of articles in this publication, please contact the Commercial Reprints Department, Elsevier Inc., 360 Park Avenue South, New York, New York 10010-1710. Tel. (212) 633-3813, Fax: (212) 462-1935, E-mail: reprints@elsevier.com.

Clinics in Laboratory Medicine (ISSN 0272-2712) is published quarterly by Elsevier Inc., 360 Park Avenue South, New York, NY 10010-1710. Months of issue are March, June, September, and December. Business and Editorial offices: 1600 John F. Kennedy Blvd., Suite 1800, Philadelphia, PA 19103-2899. Periodicals postage paid at NewYork, NY and additional mailing offices. Subscription prices are $240.00 per year (US individuals), $382.00 per year (US institutions), $128.00 (US students), $291.00 per year (Canadian individuals), $483.00 per year (foreign institutions), $176.00 (foreign students). Foreign air speed delivery is included in all *Clinics* subscription prices. All prices are subject to change without notice. POSTMASTER: Send address changes to *Clinics in Laboratory Medicine,* Elsevier Health Sciences Division, Subscription Customer Service, 3251 Riverport Lane, Maryland Heights, MO 63043. **Customer Service: 1-800-654-2452 (US). From outside of the US and Canada, call 1-314-447-8871. Fax: 1-314-447-8029. E-mail: journalscustomerservice-usa@elsevier.com (for print support) or journalsonlinesupport-usa@elsevier.com (for online support).**

Clinics in Laboratory Medicine is covered in *EMBASE/Exerpta Medica, MEDLINE/PubMed (Index Medicus), Cinahl, Current Contents/Clinical Medicine, BIOSIS* and *ISI/BIOMED.*

Printed and bound by CPI Group (UK) Ltd, Croydon, CR0 4YY

Transferred to Digital Print 2012

Contributors

GUEST EDITOR

MICHAEL G. BISSELL, MD, PhD, MPH
Professor of Pathology, The Ohio State University; Director of Clinical Chemistry and Toxicology, Wexner Medical Center at the Ohio State University, Columbus, Ohio

AUTHORS

YASH PAL AGRAWAL, MBBS, PhD
Department of Pathology and Laboratory Medicine, Weill Cornell Medical College, New York, New York

MICHAEL G. BISSELL, MD, PhD, MPH
Professor of Pathology, The Ohio State University; Director of Clinical Chemistry and Toxicology, Wexner Medical Center at the Ohio State University, Columbus, Ohio

STEVEN W. COTTEN, PhD, DABCC
Department of Pathology and Laboratory Medicine, University of North Carolina at Chapel Hill, Chapel Hill, North Carolina

GREGORY G. DAVIS, MD, MSPH
Professor, Forensic Division, Department of Pathology, University of Alabama at Birmingham; Associate Coroner/Medical Examiner, Jefferson County Coroner/Medical Examiner Office, Birmingham, Alabama

DONALD L. FREDERICK, PhD, FACB
Pathology Department, Peoria Tazewell Pathology Group, Peoria, Illinois

ROY R. GERONA, PhD
Research Scientist, Department of Laboratory Medicine, University of California, San Francisco; San Francisco General Hospital, San Francisco, California

GLYNNIS B. INGALL, MD, PhD
Associate Professor, Department of Pathology, University of New Mexico Health Sciences Center, Albuquerque, New Mexico

TAI KWONG, PhD, DABCC
Department of Pathology and Laboratory Medicine, University of Rochester, Rochester, New York

BARBARAJEAN MAGNANI, PhD, MD, FCAP
Department of Pathology and Laboratory Medicine, Tufts Medical Center, Boston, Massachusetts

STACY E.F. MELANSON, MD, PhD
Assistant Professor, Department of Pathology, Brigham and Women's Hospital, Boston, Massachusetts

HANNA RENNERT, PhD
Department of Pathology and Laboratory Medicine, Weill Cornell Medical College, New York, New York

ALAN H.B. WU, PhD
Professor, Department of Laboratory Medicine, University of California, San Francisco; Chief, Clinical Chemistry Division, San Francisco General Hospital, San Francisco, California

JOHN F. WYMAN, PhD
Chief Toxicologist, Toxicology Department, Cuyahoga County Medical Examiner's Office, Cleveland, Ohio

HOI-YING ELSIE YU, PhD
Director, Toxicology and Point-of-Care Testing, and Associate Director, Chemistry, Department of Laboratory Medicine, Geisinger Health System, Danville, Pennsylvania

Contents

metabolism. Liver enzymes, carbohydrate deficient transferrin and mean corpuscular volume are discussed as examples of indirect markers of alcohol use. Commentary on the direct ethanol markers includes the following: acetaldehyde adducts, ethyl glucuronide, ethyl sulfate, phosphatidylethanol and fatty acids ethyl esters.

Drug abusers have access to new, more potent compounds that evade existing laws by virtue of their novel chemical structures. These drugs are available for purchase at stores and over the internet. The drugs are not illegal because they are so new that laws have not yet been passed to ban them. These drugs are leading to emergency department visits for cardiovascular, neurologic, and psychiatric complications. Standard drug screens are not designed to detect these new substances. The internet provides access to drugs for substance abusers but also provides physicians speed of access to the habits of substance abusers.

"Bath salts" has attracted young adults primarily due to its stimulatory and hallucinogenic effects akin to amphetamines and cocaine. Although other designer amines have been incorporated to newer generation "bath salts", synthetic cathinones remain to be their major component. This article discusses our current understanding of the chemistry and metabolism of synthetic cathinones. It also presents a comprehensive review of the most recent laboratory analyses done on this class of compounds in drug products and biological samples.

Substance abuse is a significant problem in the United States, with cocaine, marijuana, alcohol and heroin as the most commonly abused drugs. This article focuses on urine drug testing to evaluate potential drug abuse or overdose in the emergent care setting using qualitative immunoassays. Discussion is included regarding the principles of how to validate qualitative immunoassays; how to decide on appropriate specimen type, test menu and cutoff; the limitations of immunoassays; how to communicate test results to clinicians; and use of urine drug testing at point of care.

> Drug testing in newborns comes with analytical, therapeutic, and legal issues, and interpretation of results may be left to physicians, nurses, or social services workers. The unique analytical and legal caveats pose a variety of challenges and therapeutic issues. Positive drug screening results can allow for proper medical management of withdrawal symptoms for certain drug classes. Legal implications and involvement of social services for assessment of child safety surround positive urine or meconium drug samples. Because laboratory results can potentially remove newborns from their biological parents, the caveats and limitations of drug testing in this population are of utmost importance.

> Most toxicology testing involves serum, blood, or urine. Sampling from a site of action such as nerve endings or receptors on cells is not usually available, so often blood is used. Plasma and serum are logical sources to monitor without the interference of red cells. Other types of specimens may be tested and may even be required. Most of such testing has become possible as a result of newer instrumentation. Many of these alternative specimens have very low concentrations of the drugs, drug metabolites, or other toxins. Liquid chromatography–tandem mass spectrometry has allowed testing of these alternative specimens.

> The principles and procedures employed in a modern forensic toxicology lab are detailed in this review. Aspects of Behavioral and Postmortem toxicology, including certification of analysts and accreditation of labs, chain of custody requirements, typical testing services provided, rationale for specimen selection, and principles of quality assurance are discussed. Interpretation of toxicology results in postmortem specimens requires the toxicologist and pathologist to be cognizant of drug-drug interactions, drug polymorphisms and pharmacogenomics, the gross signs of toxic pathology, postmortem redistribution, confirmation of systemic toxicity in suspected overdoses, the possibility of developed tolerance, and the effects of decomposition on drug concentration.

> Pharmacogenomics is a useful tool in clinical toxicology for characterizing many gene polymorphisms associated with different pharmacokinetics or pharmacodynamics of exogenously administered drugs. These genetic variants may determine ranges of variation in such fundamental aspects as drug-metabolizing enzymes, drug transporters, drug receptors, or targets of drug action. Toxicologically significant drugs for which the FDA has required the manufacturer to identify relevant pharmacogenomics markers on the label include carisoprodol, citalopram, codeine, and risperidone. For personalized medicine, combining pharmacogenomics testing with therapeutic drug monitoring may allow the identification of individuals who need lower or higher doses, or even a different drug.

> Clinical toxicology laboratories and forensic toxicology laboratories operate in a highly regulated environment. This article outlines major US legal/regulatory issues and requirements relevant to accreditation of toxicology laboratories (state and local regulations are not covered in any depth). The most fundamental regulatory distinction involves the purposes for which the laboratory operates: clinical versus nonclinical. The applicable regulations and the requirements and options for operations depend most basically on this consideration, with clinical toxicology laboratories being directly subject to federal law including mandated options for accreditation and forensic toxicology laboratories being subject to degrees of voluntary or state government–required accreditation.

CLINICS IN LABORATORY MEDICINE

Preface

Toxicology Testing

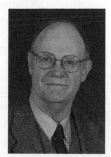

Michael G. Bissell, MD, PhD, MPH
Guest Editor

With the growth of the prescription drug epidemic, the advent of new classes of rapidly evolving designer drugs, continuing expansion of the mainstream illicit drug trade, and widespread adoption of per se drug and alcohol limits under state laws, the demand for clinical and forensic testing for drugs-of-abuse has never been greater. In this volume, the contributors have provided valuable historical background as well as reviewed the latest trends in these areas.

The topics covered here move beyond those dealt with over the years in earlier *Clinics in Laboratory Medicine* editions devoted to various aspects of Toxicology. They begin with a historical perspective on the evolution of clinical toxicology/ therapeutic drug testing as we know it today in hospital- and clinic-based settings and explore the extent and context of the growing societal problem of diversion and misuse of prescription pain medications and the structuring of laboratory operations for the support of pain clinics' need to monitor compliance, as well as the newly developing field of ethanol biomarker testing.

In the area of illicit (and/or "quasi-licit") street drugs, the scope of the problem with newly emerging psychoactive compounds is dramatized and then explored in more detail in the case of the "bath salt" (synthetic cathenone) phenomenon.

There follow some important methodological updates on drugs-of-abuse immunoassay methodology, testing of neonatal specimens, and a variety of other different body fluid specimen matrices finding increasing use in this field, as well as a general review of methods and procedures specific to forensic and postmortem testing and a glimpse of the future in which pharmacogenetics will surely eventually have an impact.

Clin Lab Med 32 (2012) xi–xii
http://dx.doi.org/10.1016/j.cll.2012.07.011
0272-2712/12/$ – see front matter © 2012 Elsevier Inc. All rights reserved.

Finally, since the practicality of all clinical and forensic drug testing is that it takes place in one of the most highly regulated environments of just about any field, an overview of this array of regulations is provided.

Michael G. Bissell, MD, PhD, MPH
Department of Pathology
The Ohio State University
4173 Graves Hall
333 West 10th Avenue
Columbus OH 43210, USA
Wexner Medical Center at the Ohio State University
4173 Graves Hall
333 West 10th Avenue
Columbus, OH 43210, USA

E-mail address:
Michael.Bissell@osumc.edu

Overview of Progress in Clinical Toxicology Testing

Donald L. Frederick, PhD[a], Michael G. Bissell, MD, PhD, MPH[b,c],*

KEYWORDS

- Poisoning • Therapeutic drug monitoring • Thin layer chromatography
- Immunoassay • High-performance liquid chromatography
- Liquid chromatography-tandem mass spectrometry

KEY POINTS

- Clinical Toxicology testing has evolved from its origins in support of the workups of toxic exposures to include therapeutic drug monitoring and drugs-of-abuse testing.
- Therapeutic drug monitoring developed out of the need to prevent and treat overdoses resulting from clinical use of potentially toxic drugs with narrow therapeutic margins.
- Drugs-of-abuse testing developed as a logical extension of the therapeutic drug monitoring menu to include abused substances, whether they are therapeutic agents or "recreational" substances.
- The ideal concept of the hospital drug screen is that blood or urine specimens are simultaneously tested for presence or concentration of multiple substances.
- The chemical methodologies utilized in the evolution of hospital drug screens have included thin layer chromatography, immunoassay, high-performance liquid chromatography, and mass spectrometry.

EVOLUTION OF THE CONCEPT OF CLINICAL TOXICOLOGY TESTING

The clinical laboratory's role in the treatment of poisoned patients in the hospital or clinic setting has evolved over the last 50 years as the scope of what is included in the workup of suspected "poisoning" has steadily broadened and physician training in toxicology has evolved. Originally, the physicians most often involved in evaluating and treating such patients were family physicians or hospital-based generalists. This began to change somewhat with the development of the field of emergency medicine.

The authors have nothing to disclose.

[a] Pathology Department, Peoria Tazewell Pathology Group, 221 NE Glen Oak Avenue, Peoria, IL 61636, USA; [b] Department of Pathology, The Ohio State University, 4173 Graves Hall, 333 West 10th Avenue, Columbus OH 43210, USA; [c] Wexner Medical Center at the Ohio State University, 4173 Graves Hall, 333 West 10th Avenue, Columbus, OH 43210, USA

* Department of Pathology, The Ohio State University, 4173 Graves Hall, 333 West 10th Avenue, Columbus, OH 43210.

E-mail address: Michael.Bissell@osumc.edu

Clin Lab Med 32 (2012) 353–359

http://dx.doi.org/10.1016/j.cll.2012.06.001
labmed.theclinics.com

The first Department of Emergency Medicine at a US medical school was founded in 1971 at the University of Southern California. Then, in 1979, the Accreditation Council for Graduate Medical Education (ACGME)-approved medical specialty of Emergency Medicine was formally initiated.

Poisoning cases were for many years mainly thought of as being narrowly limited to exposures involving toxic compounds, both naturally occurring (eg, venoms, plant toxins, metals) and industrial (eg, solvents, gases, metals). Early clinical laboratory support of these workups involved very simple tests that could aid in defining the treatment of toxicity, for example, the analysis of carboxyhemoglobin in blood to recognize and aid in the treatment of carbon monoxide poisoning. As a manual spectrophotometric procedure, the test was available initially only at larger, usually academic, medical facilities. As instruments were developed by various manufacturers, automated or semiautomated co-oximeters became more widely available to all hospitals supporting emergency treatments.

THERAPEUTIC DRUG MONITORING

As pharmaceuticals evolved, however, the proportion of poisoned patients presenting with drug overdoses escalated, resulting in the need for clinical laboratory data on drug concentrations as a basis for dose adjustment or drug removal, and this gave rise to the field of therapeutic drug monitoring. Initially, the chemical procedures needed to provide such support were complex and time consuming, with availability limited to larger academic institutions. For example, the monitoring of phenytoin was a complex multistep chemical redox reaction with photometric measurement, each specimen requiring an extraction with evaporation of the extract followed by several steps culminating in a final coupling with Bratton Marshall reagent, followed by spectrophotometric measurement of the resulting color development. The clinical demand for faster turnaround times on such testing resulted in the development of new generations of automated methods.

Several clinical premises underlie this field of therapeutic drug monitoring (TDM), namely, that certain drugs (especially the 20 or more that are near-universally routinely monitored) have:

- Narrow therapeutic ranges
- Significant (but often clinically unapparent) toxicities at supratherapeutic concentrations
- Little or no effect at subtherapeutic concentrations (again often clinically unapparent)
- Significant variation in blood drug concentration with identical doses.

Phenytoin and digoxin are classic examples of TDM-monitored drugs meeting these criteria.

Additional indications for TDM are:

- Suspected toxicity based on clinical observations (may be caused by disease or drug)
- Inadequate clinically apparent therapeutic response
- Concern with patient compliance
- Monitoring of changes in dose
- Monitoring of changes resulting from drug–drug interactions when additional drugs are added to the patient's medications.

Currently, the menu available in the clinical laboratory for TDM testing changes depending on availability of test kits and the drugs in use by current physicians and pharmaceutical companies. For automated platforms from various companies, there is a range of 13 to 25 assays available. For laboratories that have advanced equipment, such as liquid chromatography-tandem mass spectrometry (LC/MS/MS), additional assays may be added. The immunosuppressant drugs are the latest new class of drugs added to the list of those requiring TDM. Assays for these drugs are available by both LC/MS/MS and immunoassay with advantages and disadvantages with each method.

DRUGS-OF-ABUSE TESTING

The "recreational" or "sacramental" use of substances to intentionally alter mood or consciousness has occurred throughout human history. While this has, of course, long been true of a variety of naturally occurring substances subjected to relatively simple physical and chemical manipulation (eg, alcohol, tobacco, hemp, coca, opium), in more recent times, synthetic chemicals have increasingly been included. These comprise compounds that are both licit therapeutic drugs (principally, stimulants, analgesics, and sedatives) and illicit "street" drugs (principally, hallucinogens). Any of these substances can potentially give rise to signs and symptoms (behavioral as well as physical) of overdose and thus be the occasion for medical testing. In addition, testing for presence or concentrations of these substances has become important in the treatment of dependence and the monitoring of compliance or withdrawal.

With the advent of the Enzyme-Multiplied Immunoassay Technique (EMIT) technology for measuring therapeutic drugs, it was a natural progression to apply this technology to measuring "drugs of abuse." One of the first mass testing efforts was promoted by the US military as a result of heroin use in the soldiers in Vietnam. This effort was closely followed in the late 1980s by corporate America's desire to test persons for drugs of abuse as a condition of employment. As these tests became available on automated chemistry analyzers, testing on admission to emergency departments was begun to assure the treating physician that the patient did not have any of these drugs present that had the potential to influence diagnosis or interfere with treatment.

Historically, drugs-of-abuse testing began with 6 classes of drugs: amphetamines, opiates, barbiturates, cocaine metabolite, cannabinoids, and ethyl alcohol. Soon, testing for benzodiazepines, propoxyphene, phencyclidine, and methaqualone was available. Later tests for methadone, ecstasy, and LSD were added. Recent additions include buprenorphine and ketamine for specific populations. New drugs of abuse increase daily with synthetic cannabinoids as a recent class of drugs to which kit manufacturers have responded by developing a new kit that at least reacts with a few drugs in this class.[1]

EVOLUTION OF THE HOSPITAL DRUG SCREEN

The possibility of simultaneously testing for the presence of any of multiple drugs has always been theoretically attractive to emergency room physicians faced with treating cases involving suspected ingestions of unknown substances. The capability of the hospital or clinic laboratory to actually deliver such a service has been elusive, however. Nonetheless, the pursuit of such capability continues. When the primary clinical task for drug screening is identifying substances that have been previously ingested or injected, urine has historically been the specimen of choice. It is easy to obtain noninvasively in relatively large quantities, and most drugs and their metabolites (which aid the identification process) are excreted into it. However, a urine specimen lacks quantitative information that may be needed in treatment. Historically, procedures begin with differential extraction of acidic, neutral, and basic compounds followed by the main analytical challenge of separation and identification. The separation technique of thin layer chromatography (TLC), developed in the 1950s, is one in which a sheet of glass, plastic, or aluminum foil is coated with a thin layer of adsorbent material, usually silica gel, aluminium oxide, or cellulose (blotter paper), known as the *stationary phase*. After the sample has been applied to the plate, a solvent or solvent mixture, known as the *mobile phase*, is applied to the plate via capillary action. Spatial separation of sample analytes is effected by their differential mobile phase solubility coupled with differences in their affinity for the solid phase. Detection of the separated analytes is typically ultraviolet (UV)/visual and qualitative.

TLC has had a significant impact on the problem of identification of known and unknown substances in biological fluids. TLC applications in the identification of drugs first appeared in the 1960s, and, by 1972, TLC extraction and separation procedures for urine drugs were utilized to identify a wide range of drugs. With the introduction of a standardized set of reagents and chromatography procedures in the 1980s, TLC became the basis of drug screening methods for many hospital and clinic laboratories[2–4] and are still in use (with some modifications) in some laboratories.[5] This methodology requires little capital investment and is relatively easy to perform, but the quality of results is technique dependent and interpretation can be very subjective.

The advent of immunoassay technology fundamentally changed the way toxicology laboratories handled drug screens. The limited drug screen came into use in addition to (or in place of) the comprehensive screen. Immunoassay companies developed screens for drug classes (ie, amphetamines, benzodiazepines) based on the interaction of an antibody developed against one member of the drug class with some cross reactivity to other drugs in the class. Many hospital laboratories responded by instituting series of these immunoassay screens. The main advantages are (1) the ability to automate these procedures, reducing turnaround times, and (2) the opportunity to utilize less highly trained technologists. Some larger hospital laboratories began to have these immunoassays available with immediate turnaround (ie, as STAT assays) while having the TLC or other comprehensive screen as a follow-up (not STAT) procedure when additional information was needed.

The next stage in the evolution of the comprehensive drug screen was the advent and combination of 2 fundamental technologic advances: (1) the development and use of the concept of the *drug library*— a database of chemical spectral identifications of a wide range of compounds that can be compared with the output of the detector on a chemical separation device, and (2) the application of automation to the problem of comprehensive drug screening.

The initial work on the first of these advances occurred in the early 1970s in laboratories of the National Institute of Standards and Technology.[6] This was applied and extended to drug identification in suspected overdose cases in 1971 by Law and colleagues.[7]

Then in the 1990s, the Bio-Rad company introduced the first automated emergency drug profiling system, the BioRad REMEDi, a serially linked multicolumn high-performance liquid chromatographic system coupled to a library database of UV spectra for more than 900 drugs and their metabolites.[8] High-performance liquid chromatography is a form of liquid chromatography that utilizes small-size columns (typically 250 mm or shorter and 4.6 mm interior diameter or smaller) packed with stationary phases consisting of different types of smaller sorbent particles and having mobile phase pumped through them at high pressures. Sample analytes are separated temporally, exiting the column past a detector capable of providing their characteristic retention times and area counts reflecting the amount of each, plus additional information (ie, UV/visual spectroscopic data), if so equipped. With the REMEDi system, urine specimens required no pretreatment and were automatically introduced into the system, which separated the constituent peaks and compared their UV spectra with the drug library and produced a probability match. This system quickly became the mainstay of emergency drug screening in many hospital and clinic laboratories and was relied on by them for many years. Unfortunately, the manufacturer, Bio-Rad, discontinued support of the system in December of 2007 without recommendation as to an alternative,[9] even though more extensive UV libraries had been published.[10]

Methods based on liquid chromatographic separation coupled with highly selective mass spectrometric detection have begun to fill the void left by the REMEDi.[11] Prominent among these are liquid chromatography-mass spectrometry (LC/MS) and LC/MS/MS, which (unlike the gas chromatographic separation methods in use for a number of individual drug analyses) potentially provide the capability to directly analyze aqueous samples containing multiple hydrophilic analytes that are thermolabile and nonvolatile. LC/MS-based drug screening detection methods are of 2 basic types: (1) those based on comparisons against instrument-specific libraries, and (2) those representing systematic screening against libraries of ultimate molecular mass standards.

In the first approach (exemplified by routine practice in coauthor's laboratory), mass spectrometers are used to generate information-rich product ion spectra, which are compared with libraries of reference mass spectra previously recorded on the same or similar instruments, that is, instruments based on triple quadrupole, ion trap, or hybrid mass spectrometer technology.

Quadrupoles are sets of 4 parallel metal rods used to accelerate ions differentially and separate them spatially according to their mass-to-charge ratios. In triple electromagnetic quadrupole configurations, the first (Q_1) and third (Q_3) quadrupoles act in this way as mass filters, and the middle (q_2) quadrupole is used as a collision cell in which an inert gas is used for collision-induced dissociation of selected parent ion(s) originating from Q_1. Subsequent fragments are passed through to Q_3 where they may be filtered or fully scanned. This process allows for the study of fragments (daughter ions) that are crucial in structural elucidation, providing great specificity of identification.

Ion traps are combinations of electric or magnetic fields that capture ions in a specific region. They are conceptually similar to quadrupoles but direct ions to oscillate in or around a single focus, rather than along a linear axis. Ions so entrapped can be detected after ejection from the trap or by virtue of the oscillating current they induce in a detection circuit.

Hybrid mass spectrometers combine both triple quadrupole and ion trap configurations to combine specificity and full scan MS/MS sensitivity to provide simultaneous qualitative and quantitative results.

There are many instrument-specific variables involved in the operation of hybrid LC/MS/MS instruments such that the libraries used for drug screening using this approach must also be derived in an instrument-specific fashion.

The second approach (as exemplified by work at the University of California, San Francisco[12]) is based on high-resolution mass spectrometry with benchtop time-of-flight mass spectrometers, in which compounds are identified by comparison of accurate masses as measured in the sample with accurate (instrument-independent) mass databases of toxicologically relevant compounds.

In time-of-flight mass spectrometry, an ion's mass-to-charge ratio is determined via a time measurement. Ions are accelerated by an electric field of known strength, resulting in every ion with the same charge having the same kinetic energy, and each ion's velocity then depending on its mass-to-charge ratio (heavier particles being slower).[13] The times that individual ions take to reach a detector at a precisely known distance are highly accurately measured by means of a time-to-digital converter or a fast analog-to-digital converter, captured in discrete time "bins." Hundreds of these measurements, in turn, are summed into histograms, which constitute the peaks of mass spectra. Molecular masses determined in this way are instrument independent and can be directly compared with libraries of molecular masses that are fundamentally accurate. Each new generation of instrument increases the accuracy of the molecular weight determination and thus narrows the selection of possible molecules for a given peak identification. Current instruments determine mass to 2 parts per million accuracy, which translates to an atomic mass unit error of only 0.0008 at a molecular weight of 400. The use of these new techniques is being applied to both targeted and nontargeted screens. Targeted screens are developed for specific types of clinical situations, such as seizure panel, synthetic cannabinoid panel, and CYP 2D6 panel. Nontargeted panels are the typical drug screens based on historical knowledge of the drugs of abuse and drugs involved in overdoses. An added feature of this instrumentation is that a quantitative serum screen is possible with turnaround times of 90 to 120 minutes.

Although these mass spectrometric–based methods arguably represent the current state of the art in terms of discrimination and (ultimate) accuracy, they are not parts of high-throughput fully automated specimen flow or interpretation in most clinical toxicology laboratories in which they are used, and thus turnaround time remains a challenge. Furthermore, they represent a major increase in operating expense, both in terms of the size of the capital investment required and the skill level of the operators needed to produce results. Yet, the challenge and pursuit of the ultimate goal of achieving a comprehensive real-time drug screen continues.

REFERENCES

1. Randox Toxicology Corprate Website. Available at: http://www.randoxtoxicology.com/Products/Elisa-p-50. Accessed June 14, 2012.
2. Jarvie DR, Simpson D. Drug screening: evaluation of the Toxi-Lab TLC System. Ann Clin Biochem 1986;23:76–84.
3. Gaenshirt H, Malzacher A. [Thin-layer chromatography in drug analysis]. Arch Pharm 1960;293/65:925–32 [in German].
4. Baeumler J, Rippstein S. [Thin-layer chromatography as a rapid method for the analysis of drugs]. Plast Reconstr Surg 1961;36:382–8 [in German].
5. Kaistha KK, Jaffe JH. TLC techniques for identification of narcotics, barbiturates, and CNS stimulants in a drug abuse urine screening program. J Pharm Sci 1972;61:679–89.
6. Heller SR, Fales HM, Milne GW, et al. Letter: mass spectral search system. Biomed Mass Spectrom 1974;1:207–8.
7. Law NC, Aandahl V, Fales HM, et al. Identification of dangerous drugs by mass spectrometry. Clin Chim Acta 1971;32:221–8.
8. Kalasinsky KS, Schaefer T, Binder SR. Forensic application of an automated drug-profiling system. J Anal Toxicol 1995;19:412–8.
9. Maurer H, Peters F. Towards high-throughput drug screening using mass spectrometry. Ther Drug Monit 2005;27:686–8.

10. Herzler M, Herre S, Pragst F. Selectivity of substance identification by HPLC-DAD in toxicological analysis using a UV spectra library of 2682 compounds. J Anal Toxicol 2003;27:233–42.
11. Maurer HH. Current role of liquid chromatography-mass spectrometry in clinical and forensic toxicology. Anal Bioanal Chem 2007;388:1315–25.
12. Gerona RRL, Wu AHB. Clinical Uility of an LC-MS/TOF seizure panel in emergency department's seizure patients. Clin Chem 2010;56(6 Suppl):A245.
13. Cotter RJ. Time-of-flight mass spectrometry. Columbus (OH): American Chemical Society; 1994.

The Prescription Drug Abuse Epidemic

Hoi-Ying Elsie Yu, PhD

KEYWORDS

- Drug diversion • Opioids • Benzodiazepines • Stimulants

KEY POINTS

- In the United States, diversion of prescription drugs to nonmedical use has grown to epidemic proportions, with only cannabis exceeding them among categories of illicit drug use.
- The three most widely diverted classes of prescription drugs currently are the opioids, central nervous system (CNS) depressants (eg, benzodiazepines), and CNS stimulants (eg, amphetamine, dextroamphetamine, and methylphenidate).
- In the first decade of the 21st century, U.S. retail sales of opioid drugs more than doubled, with prescriptions increasing from 76 to 210 million.
- Similar increases were seen during this period among the commonly prescribed benzodiazepine tranquilizers including alprazolam (Xanax), diazepam (Valium), lorazepam (Ativan), clonazepam (Klonopin), and temazepam (Restoril).
- Stimulants were likewise prescribed in record numbers for treatment of attention-deficit/hyperactivity disorder, including amphetamine/dextroamphetamine (Adderall, Dexedrine) and methylphenidate (Concerta, Ritalin).

In the United States, the nonmedical use of prescription drugs is the second most common illicit drug use, behind only marijuana.[1] According to the United States Centers for Disease Control and Prevention (CDC), more than 36,000 people died as a result of a drug poisoning in 2008, representing an increase of 138% when compared to the approximately 15,000 deaths in 1998.[2] Of these deaths, more than 40% involved prescription opioids.[2] The number of deaths from prescription overdose is believed to have surpassed the combined number of deaths from cocaine, heroin, and methamphetamine.[3] The Report by the Drug Abuse Warning Network (DAWN) on the estimated number of emergency department (ED) visits related to drug abuse further illustrates the problem.[4] In 2009, there were more than 1,000,000 drug-related ED visits, an increase of 101% as compared to 2004. From 2004 to 2009,

The author has nothing to disclose.
Department of Laboratory Medicine, Geisinger Health System, 100 North Academy Avenue, Danville, PA 17822-0131, USA
E-mail address: heyu@geisinger.edu

the estimated ED visits involving the nonmedical use of (1) prescription opioids increased by 141% (from 172,700 to 416,500 visits); (2) benzodiazepines increased by 118% (from 143,500 to 312,900 visits); (3) stimulants such as amphetamine-dextroamphetamine and methylphenidate increased by 187% (from 4700 to 13,600 visits).[4] In addition to mortality and morbidity, this has also resulted in loss of productivity. Furthermore, prescription drug diversion poses a public safety threat. According to the National Drug Treatment Assessment, more state and law enforcement agencies associated property crime and violent crime with prescription diversion.[3] The estimated cost of illicit drug use was estimated to be more than $193 billion in 2007.[3] This includes the cost of crimes, health care, and productivity loss.[3]

This article discusses the abuse issues with three of the most widely abused prescription drugs: opioids, central nervous system (CNS) depressants (eg, benzodiazepines), and stimulants (eg, amphetamine-dextroamphetamine and methylphenideate) in the United States.

OPIOIDS
Intended Medical Use

Opioids are analgesics that bind to opioid receptors most commonly used for pain relief.[5–7] The drugs can also be used as antitussive and antidiarrheal agents. Some of the commonly prescribed opioids include hydrocodone (eg, Vicodin), hydromorphone (eg, Dilaudid), oxycodone (eg, Percocet), oxymorphone, fentanyl (eg, Duragesic), methadone, buprenorphine (eg, suboxone), morphine, and codeine. Of these, methadone and buprenorphine are more commonly used to treat opioid dependence.[7] Between 1997 and 2007, the retail sales of opioids more than doubled, with 126.5 million grams sold in 2007.[8] From 1991 to 2010, the total number of opioid prescriptions increased from 76 million to 210 million.[9] This reflected changes in physicians' practice, as opioids are increasingly used to treat chronic pain, in addition to acute and postsurgical pain, and for palliative care.[8] The increased pain awareness from both the providers and patients has also resulted in more pain prescriptions. The United States may have the most serious issue on this, as the United States accounts for the consumption of approximately 80% of the world's supply of opioids, even though only 4.6% of the world's population lives in the United States.[8]

Abuse Trend

Between 1999 and 2008, deaths associated with the use of opioids have increased from approximately 4000 to 14,800, a rate that surpasses deaths involving other drugs.[2] Of these, more deaths occurred among men than women.[8,10] The majority of the 14,800 deaths were associated with natural and semisynthetic opioids such as morphine, hydrocodone, and oxycodone.[2] In 2008, these opioids were involved in more than 9100 deaths, more than double the 2700 deaths reported in 1999.[2] Methadone was associated with approximately 5000 deaths in 2008, more than six times of those in 1999.[2] Of particular concern is that methadone-related deaths substantially outnumbered those associated with other opioids when adjusted for the number of prescriptions issued.[11] Methadone accounted for less than 5% of total opioids prescribed, but a third of all opioid-related deaths were associated with it.[11] Deaths involving other synthetic opioids (excluding methadone) such as fentanyl showed a steady increase, totaling approximately 2300 in 2008, more than triple the approximately 700 deaths in 1999.[2]

The rates of ED visits showed a similar trend. In 2009, approximately 288,700 ED visits were related to natural and semisynthetic opioids, more than double that of 2004 (**Fig. 1**).[4] The majority of these deaths involved oxycodone (148,400 visits) and

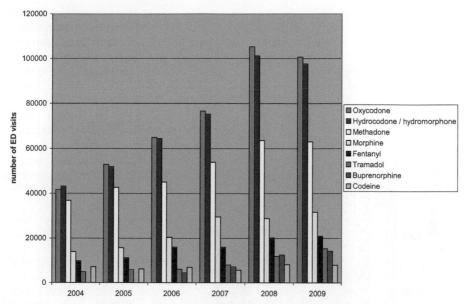

Fig. 1. ED visits relating to opioids. (*From* Substance Abuse and Mental Health Services Administration. Drug Abuse Warning Network, 2009: National estimates of drug-related emergency department visits. HHS Publication No. (SMA) 11-4659, DAWN Series D-35. Rockville (MD): Substance Abuse and Mental Health Services Administration, 2011.)

hydrocodone (86,300 visits) (see **Fig. 1**).[4] Methadone was involved in 63,000 visits and fentanyl was involved in 20,900 visits (see **Fig. 1**).[4] ED visits related to buprenorphine were also on the rise, with 14,300 in 2008, more than triple that in 2006 (see **Fig. 1**). However, some caution that the increased number of buprenorphine-related ED visits or death may be due not to buprenorphine, but to the underlying drug (eg, heroin) addiction problem.[12]

Some groups are more likely to overdose on prescription opioids than others. According to the CDC, whites and American Indians are more prone to overdose.[10] Middle-aged adults have one of the highest overdose rates.[10] Overdose is two times more likely to happen in rural areas than in big cities.[10] The states that have higher sales of opioids per person (eg, Florida and West Virginia) also tend to have more deaths from opioid overdose.[10] Opioid abusers are not the only group at risk for overdose and death. Patients who are prescribed with high or frequent dosage are also at substantial risk, especially if a sedative is also prescribed.[11,12]

According to the 2010 National Survey on Drug Use and Health, there were an estimated 5.1 million nonmedical users of pain relievers (**Fig. 2**).[1] Prevalence of opioid abuse among American Indians (1 in 10) is two times that of whites (1 in 20) and three times that of blacks (1 in 30).[10] The direct health care costs total approximately $72.5 billion annually as a result of this high prevalence of opioid abuse.[10] Among youths and young adults, the prevalence of prescription opioids misuse has remained relatively stable since 2002, ranging from 6.2% to 7.7% for youths aged 12 to 17, and 11.1% to 12.4% for young adults aged 18 to 25.[1] However, females aged 12 to 17 were more likely to be opioid abusers than males in the same age (3.0% vs 2.0%).[1] Since 2002, there were more than 2.0 million new users who abuse prescription opioids each year.[1] From 2002 to 2010, the rate of opioid dependence has increased

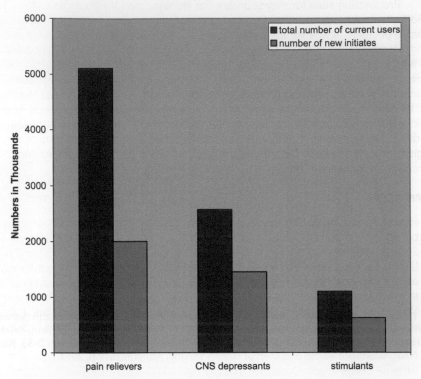

Fig. 2. Nonmedical use of prescription drugs in 2010. (*From* Substance Abuse and Mental Health Services Administration. Results from the 2010 National Survey on Drug Use and Health: summary of national findings, NSDUH Series H-41, HHS Publication No. (SMA) 11-4658. Rockville (MD): Substance Abuse and Mental Health Services Administration; 2011.)

from 0.4% to 0.6% of the population, resulting in an increase from 936,000 to 1,400,000 people.[1] About 57% of these were aged 26 or older, and the other one third were aged 18 to 25.[1] Despite the relatively steady prevalence of opioid abuse in recent years, the number of people who entered treatment programs has more than doubled from 2002 to 2010, with approximately 66% aged 26 or older, and approximately 26% aged 18 to 25.[1]

Misuse Motive

Opioids have long been an attractive recreational drug owing to their ability to induce a feeling of euphoria.[5] As tolerance to the drug develops, abusers seek higher dose or more potent drug to reach the "high." At the same time, users want to avoid the unpleasant withdrawal symptoms such as inability to sleep, anxiety, chills, runny nose, sweating, muscle twitching, muscle ache, and agitation.[5] This ensures further craving for the drugs.

Furthermore, many perceive prescription opioid abuse as safer, less stigmatizing and less illegal when compare to other illicit drugs.[13] The use of prescription opioids also may appear to be a better alternative than heroin,[13] in overcoming heroin withdrawal or tolerance. Fourteen times more people tried prescription opioids than heroin for the first time in 2010.[1]

The increase of prescription use of opioids has likely led to more drug addiction and dependence problems. From 1999 to 2010, four times more opioids are being sold to pharmacies, hospitals, and physicians' offices. As the number of patients who are on opioids increases, so does the number of people at risk of becoming addicted to the drugs. Although there are no solid data on the likelihood of becoming addicted to the drug after legitimate medical use, news reports have described patients who became addicted to opioids during the course of treatment.[14] Studies have shown that patients are more likely to become long-term opioid users if they were prescribed with an opioid within 7 days of surgery, compared with those who received no opioid prescription.[15] Thus, opioid dependence appears to be associated with exposure to the drug, regardless of whether or not the initial exposure is legitimate. In addition, 15% to 23% of patients with chronic pain appeared to meet criteria as substance abusers,[16] and many use opioids as an escape from social and financial stress.

The increase of prescription use of opioids has also increased their supply and accessibility. According to the 2010 National Survey on Drug Use and Health,[1] approximately 17% of abusers indicated that they obtained their opioids via prescriptions from a physician. In 2010, more than 70% obtained their opioids from their relatives and friends, mostly for free.[1] About 80% of the friends and relatives obtained their drugs from only one physician.[1] Relatively few (about 4.4%) opioids abusers bought their supply from a drug dealer or other stranger or over the Internet.[1] Moreover, the increase of opioid inventories in retail pharmacies likely fuels illegal drug trafficking. For example, in 2003, there were at least 6 million doses of opioids stolen from retail pharmacies.[17]

Adverse Effects

Although different opioids have various potencies with specific side effects, some common signs of opioid overdose include loss of muscle tone, confusion, bradycardia, hypotension, stupor, respiratory depression, and coma.[5–7] In severe cases, coma with respiratory depression can often result in sudden death.[5] This is particularly dangerous for users who also abuse other sedatives such as alcohol, benzodiazepines, and barbiturates, which cause further respiratory depression problems. Alcohol and/or benzodiazepines are found frequently in opioid-related deaths.[11] Users who prefer more rapid onset by injecting, smoking, or snorting are also more likely to suffer from acute respiratory depression. In addition, peripheral nerve trauma, pulmonary hypertension, and bloodborne infections (if sharing needles) are common problems associated with injecting drug users.[5] Necrosis of the intranasal structures including soft and hard palate has also been reported from snorting of opioids.[18,19]

Preventive Measures

As morbidity and mortality associated with nonmedical use of prescription opioids continues to grow, much focus has been placed on reducing the risk of opioid prescription. Many physicians use various risk assessment and treatment strategies to minimize misuse of opioids.[20]

Initial medical assessment including a thorough review of medical and prescription history, a urine drug screen, physical examination, and a psychological evaluation should be conducted for patients who are considered for opioid therapy to identify the suitability and potential risk of opioid treatment.[20] Substance abuse assessment should also be conducted to identify patients who are prone to the misuse of opioids.[20] Several of the opioid risk assessment tools have been validated and shown to be useful in identifying patients at risk: Screener and Opioid Assessment for Patients in Pain-Revised (SOAPP-R); Current Opioid Misuse Measure (COMM);

Opioid Risk Tool (ORT); Diagnosis, Intractability, Risk, and Efficacy (DIRE); Screening Instrument for Substance Abuse Potential (SISAP); and the Pain Assessment and Documentation Tool (PADT).[20] Regular use of urine toxicology screen to monitor the patients' compliance to the treatment regimen has helped identify aberrant drug-use behavior.[20] However, misinterpretation of test results can undermine the effectiveness of the drug monitoring program.[6] Opioid therapy agreement can also be used to inform/educate patients of their roles in the treatment program and clarify some of the rules that the patients need to follow to ensure effective treatment and minimize misuse.[20] For patients who have been identified at high risk of opioid abuse or have misused opioids, behavioral intervention can help minimize those risks and help the patients become compliant.[20]

Use of tamper-resistant and abuse-deterrent opioid formulations has also been shown to have varying success.[20] Tamper-resistant drugs are designed to make it difficult or unpleasant for injection or inhalation.[20] Examples include Oxecta, Remoxy, COL-003, and TQ-1017. Abuse-deterrent drugs are usually mixed with one or more antagonists or aversive agents to make them less attractive for abuse.[20] Examples include suboxone (buprenorphine with the antagonist naloxone), Embeda (morphine with the antagonist naltrexone), ELI-216 (oxycodone with the antagonist naltrexone), and Acurox (oxycodone with the aversive agent niacin).

Other programs aim to lower the risk for high-dose users. For example, there are now at least 188 local opioid overdose prevention programs nationwide since the first program started in 1996.[21] These programs provide naloxone (an opioid antagonist that is used to treat opioid overdose) and other overdose prevention services to those who use the drugs, their friends and families, as well as health care providers, homeless shelters, and other substance treatment programs.[21] They provide education on overdose risk factors, signs of opioid overdose, proper responses to an overdose, and administration of naloxone.[21] In 1995–2010, these programs had provided naloxone to approximately 53,000 people, reversing approximately 10,100 opioid overdoses.[21] A shift from methadone clinics to office-based care using buprenorphine is also thought to improve the treatment of opioid dependence.[22] First, buprenorphine appears to be safer than methadone.[7] Second, the office-based care is thought to be less stigmatizing and more accessible to all patients.[23]

In April 2011, the White House released its plan to address the opioid abuse epidemic.[24] It includes four components. First, education is needed to increase the awareness of the public and health care providers about the dangers of opioid misuse.[24] In addition, the plan requires that health care providers be trained on how to properly prescribe these drugs. In 2000, only 56% of medical residency programs required substance use disorder training.[24] Most physicians receive little guidelines on how to prescribe opioids appropriately. Evidence-base guidelines need to be developed to educate prescribers on how these drugs should be used and minimize risk and ensure proper medical use. These would include proper prescription dosage, risk evaluation, and mitigation strategy, as well as patient–provider agreements. A recent root cause analysis for opioid-related deaths found that the dose of medication might have been too high and that prescribers might not have considered reducing the prescription of other potentially dangerous medications such as benzodiazepines when opioids were used.[11] This further highlights the importance of practice guidelines.

Second, prescription drug monitoring programs need to be operational in all states to help detect and prevent diversion and abuse of prescription drugs.[24] As of June 2012, 41 states had operational programs, and 8 others had passed enacting legislation.[23] These programs are established by state legislation to track all controlled substances prescriptions, and thereby can help identify "doctor/pharmacist shoppers" and "pill mills." The data can also help health insurance programs to identify fraud and set up new policy. For example, Blue Cross Blue Shield of Massachusetts recently initiates a new preauthorization program for some of the pain medications to reduce inappropriate painkillers prescription.[25] In addition, health insurance programs can set up claims review programs to identify inappropriate use of opioids for unrelated diagnoses.[23]

Third, proper disposal of unused medication is needed to help reduce diversion because many abusers obtain their opioid supply from families and friends.[24] Currently, the Drug Enforcement Administration (DEA) is drafting such rules. The National Prescription Drug Take-Back Events in 2010 and 2011, during which where approximately 309 tons of drugs were collected nationwide, have also increased the awareness of proper drug disposal.[23]

Fourth, improvement and enforcement of legislation that outlaws "doctor shoppers" and "pill mills" are critical in cracking down illegal drug trafficking.[24] Although most states have laws against doctor shopping, only a few have laws against distributing prescription drugs with minimal medical evaluation.[23] Clear "Pain Clinic Regulation Laws" need to be defined to shut down "pill mills"[24] and prevent prescription fraud.[23] For example, as of October 1, 2010, Florida's pain clinic law requires that pain management clinics (with some exceptions) must register with the state Department of Health.[3] The Department of Health then inspects these clinics for proper operation annually. In addition, the law establishes limits that no more than 3 days' worth of pain medication can be dispensed for each patient.[3] Further, doctors are required to have extensive training in pain issues to prescribe pain medication.[3] Texas has a law that requires pain clinics be registered with the Texas Medical Board and be owned and operated by licensed medical directors.[3]

CNS DEPRESSANTS
Intended Medical Use

CNS depressants are medications that slow normal brain function, commonly used to treat anxiety disorders and insomnia. They include barbiturates, benzodiazepines, and new nonbenzodiazepine sleep medications. Barbiturates decrease synaptic transmissions by affecting the functions of glutamate and γ-aminobutyric acid (GABA) receptors, as well as calcium and chloride channels.[26] They have anxiolytic, sedative, hypnotic, anticonvulsant, and anesthetic properties.[26] Although barbiturates were once commonly used to treat sleep and anxiety disorders, benzodiazepines and other newer nonbenzodiazepine medications are now more commonly used because these drugs have safer profiles. Phenobarbital and butalbital are a few of the barbiturates that are still used, mostly as anticonvulsants or in combination with other analgesics to treat headache, respectively. Analysis by the Substance Abuse and Mental Health Services Administration (SAMHSA) and the Food and Drug Administration (FDA) showed that there has been a significant reduction in barbiturate prescriptions in recent years.[27] Based on the total number of prescriptions dispensed through the outpatient retail pharmacies, from 1998 to 2007, phenobarbital prescriptions decreased by 22% (820,000), and butalbital prescription decreased by 61% (381,000).[27]

Benzodiazepines are commonly used to treat anxiety disorders, insomnia, panic disorders, seizures, and muscle spasticity.[28] They bind to the GABA receptors, producing anxiolytic, sedative, hypnotic, anticonvulsant, and muscle relaxant properties.[28] Some of the commonly prescribed benzodiazepines include alprazolam

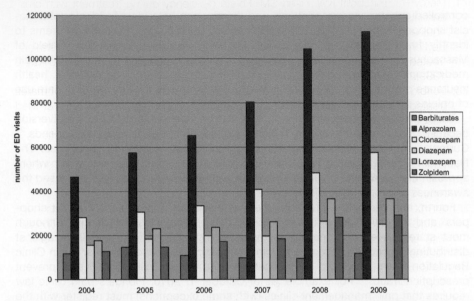

Fig. 3. ED visits related to CNS depressants. (*From* Substance Abuse and Mental Health Services Administration. Drug Abuse Warning Network, 2009: National estimates of drug-related emergency department visits. HHS Publication No. (SMA) 11-4659, DAWN Series D-35. Rockville (MD): Substance Abuse and Mental Health Services Administration, 2011.)

(Xanax), diazepam (Valium), lorazepam (Ativan), clonazepam (Klonopin), and temazepam (Restoril). From 1998 to 2007, there was a 114% increase (10.9 million) in clonazepam prescriptions, a 71% increase (17.6 million) in alprazolam, a 30% increase (1.9 million) in temazepam, a 24% increase (4.2 million) in lorazepam, and a 17% increase (2.1 million) in diazepam.[27]

Nonbenzodiazepines hypnotics, also known as "Z-drugs," include zolpidem (Ambien), zaleplon (Sonata), and eszopiclone (Lunesta). They are designed to target selective GABA receptor to aid sleeping, and may be less prone to tolerance or dependence issues.[29] According to study done by Thomson Reuters, there was a 50% increase in the use of prescription sleep aids in young adults between 1998 and 2006.[30] In 2006, two thirds of these were nonbenzodiazepine hypnotics, compared to only 41% in 1998,[30] representing an approximately140% increase of nonbenzodiazepine sleep medications prescriptions.

Abuse Trend

In 2009, at least 32.8% of ED visits were related to CNS depressants.[4] About 11,800 ED visits involved barbiturates, similar to the number in 2004 (**Fig. 3**).[4] On the other hand, ED visits involving benzodiazepines more than doubled during the same time period (see **Fig. 3**).[4] In 2009, approximately 312,900 ED visits involved benzodiazepines, where approximately 112,600 visits involved alprazolam and approximately 57,600 visits involved clonazepam (see **Fig. 3**).[4] Similarly, ED visits involving zolpidem increased from approximately 12,800 visits in 2004 to approximately 29,000 visits in 2009 (see **Fig. 3**).[4] These showed an alarming increase in the abuse of benzodiazepines and other nonbenzodiazepine sleeping aids. In addition, there was a significant increase in the involvement of alprazolam, clonazepam, and zolpidem in drug-related suicide cases since 2004, with a 148% increase for zolpidem and a 105% increase for alprazolam.[4] This further highlights the extent of misuse of these drugs. Therefore, the rest of the "CNS depressants" section focuses on benzodiazepine and nonbenzodiazepine hypnotics.

According to the 2010 National Survey on Drug Use and Health, there were an estimated 2.57 million nonmedical users of tranquilizers and sedatives (see **Fig. 2**).[1] Unfortunately, the survey did not include results on specific tranquilizers or sedatives. However, about 80% of people who abused benzodiazepines also misused other drugs, most commonly opioids.[31] Further, an estimated 3% to 41% of alcoholic persons abused benzodiazepines.[31] In 2010, there were approximately 1.4 million new users of tranquilizers and sedatives (see **Fig. 2**).[1] The mean age at which misuse of these drugs was initiated was 24 years old.[1] However, abuse in older people is probably under-recognized.[32] The prevalence of benzodiazepine prescriptions for anxiolytic and hypnotic causes in people older than the age of 65 years are significantly higher.[33] In addition, more women received prescriptions for benzodiazepines than men.[33] Yet, only one third of the prescriptions were estimated to be appropriate,[33] suggesting misuse in the other two thirds. In addition, people who are mentally or physically vulnerable are more likely to misuse these drugs.[33]

Misuse Motive

CNS depressants are subjected to abuse owing to their ability to relax anxious feelings and remove inhibitions, similar to the euphoric feeling induced by alcohol. The increase of prescription use of benzodiazepines has also led to more addiction and dependence issues. Prolonged usage of benzodiazepines results in the physical dependence of the drugs because withdrawal may result in undesirable symptoms such as insomnia, tremors, agitation, anxiety, and muscle spasms.[34]

The increases of prescriptions for benzodiazepine and nonbenzodiazepine hypnotics have also increased the availability and accessibility of these drugs, resulting in more misuse, as indicated by the increase of ED visits related to these drugs (**Fig. 3**). As with opioid abusers, most nonmedical users of these sedatives obtain their supply from a friend or relative who got the supply from legitimate prescriptions.[1] In addition, drug diversion is common.[35]

Benzodiazepines are often used in combination with opioids and/or alcohol to potentiate the euphoric effect.[31] In addition, they are used by cocaine addicts to relieve some of the side effects associated with cocaine use, for example, irritability and agitation.[31] They are also used with amphetamines or other stimulants to relieve anxiety after a binge and to induce sleep.[31,33] Prescription benzodiazepines and other nonbenzodiazepine hypnotics are also used as "date rape" drugs although flunitrazepam (Rohypnol), a benzodiazepine that is well known for this purpose, is not legal in the United States.[35] In most cases, abusers take these CNS depressants orally. However, some prefer taking them intranasally and intravenously for more potent effect.[33]

Adverse Effects

Benzodiazepine overdoses are rarely fatal if used alone. In 2010, benzodiazepines were involved in more than 80,000 poisoning cases reported to the poison centers in the United States.[36] Most of those cases also involved other abuse substances such as opioids and alcohol where benzodiazepenes likely contribute to morbidity and mortality.[11,36] Among them, more than 300 cases resulted in "major events" and 11 cases resulted in deaths.[36]

Generally, sedative drugs can cause a decline in processing speed, learning abilities, and cognitive functions.[33] In addition, these drugs increase the likelihood of accidents and injuries such as falls or driving accidents.[33] Benzodiazepine abuse can also produce disinhibitory and aggressive effects that result in violence and assault.[33] If used with alcohol and opioids, the aforementioned problems are more common and severe.[33] Although they give an initial euphoric effects, a horrifying sense of anxiety could follow during withdrawal.[34] Intravenous use of sedatives can result in peripheral nerve trauma and the likelihood of bloodborne infections increases if needles are shared.

Preventive Measures

Unlike opioids, the abuse of benzodiazepines and Z-drugs has not caught the same level of national attention in the United States. However, other countries such as the United Kingdom had expressed more concerns on the use of these sedatives with national campaigns.[33] Nevertheless, attempts have been made to reduce the prescription of benzodiazepines in the United States. For example, the development of Z-drugs is presumed to be safer in the treatment of insomnia and the number of prescriptions has increased. Selective serotonin reuptake inhibitors (SSRIs) are the preferred treatment for panic disorder according to the American Psychiatric Association's practice guideline.[37] However, SSRIs take weeks to produce any benefit. Therefore, benzodiazepines can appear more effective to patients because of their rapid onset of action.[37] In addition, benzodiazepines have shown proven efficacy for treatment of acute anxiety and generalized anxiety disorder problems[31]; therefore it is not surprising that benzodiazepines continue to be commonly used.

Most patients who are prescribed benzodiazepines for legitimate use do not abuse benzodiazepines.[33] However, for patients who have other substance abuse problem, providers may wish to choose an appropriate alternative that is less prone to abuse.[31] Therefore, it is important for clinicians to identify patients who may be at risk of abuse. A thorough review of personal and family history in addition to the medical history could be helpful.[38] Urine toxicology screen can also help identify patients who are abusing other drugs (eg, opioids) or diverting their benzodiazepine prescriptions. However, proper interpretation of urine test results could be difficult. Immunoassays that are commonly used by clinical laboratories to qualitatively screen for benzodiazepines have various sensitivity for different benzodiazepines.[28] For example, the assay by Roche can effectively screen for clonazepam but not lorazepam. Although more sensitive chromatography–mass spectrometry methods can analyze different benzodiazepines, different clinical laboratories may analyze different benzodiazepines in their testing panels. Therefore, it is important to consult the medical laboratories to have an understanding of which benzodiazepines are being analyzed. Finally, most screening tests do not currently screen for Z-drugs. Therefore, testing for those drugs usually needs to be specially requested as a send-out to reference laboratories.

Better management of cessation of use may help alleviate some of the withdrawal symptoms that lead to misuse of the drugs. Some of the strategies include gradual taper of medication and conversion to alternative medications such as benzodiazepines with slower onset of action or other GABA receptor modulators that have a higher safety profile.[33,38] Psychological treatments and cognitive–behavioral therapies may also help.[33]

According to the National Institute of Mental Health, most anxiety disorders should be treated with a combination of psychological treatments (eg, cognitive–behavioral therapies) and medications. Cognitive–behavioral therapy is also recommended for treatment of insomnia by the American Academy of Sleep Medicine's Practice Parameters.[39] However, it is not clear how many patients who received anxiolytic/sedative medications receive psychological treatments. A practical guideline that includes discussion of these nonpharmacologic treatment options could be useful to reduce anxiolytic/sedative prescriptions.[33,40]

STIMULANTS
Intended Medical Use

Stimulants are agents that can increase alertness and attention. They increase the concentration of dopamine, norepinephrine, and epinephrine in the synaptic clefts via various mechanisms, thereby enhancing synaptic transmission.[41] Their most widely recognizable therapeutic use is probably for treatment of attention-deficit/hyperactivity disorder (ADHD). Some of the commonly used medications include amphetamine/dextroamphetamine (Adderall, Dexedrine) and methylphenidate (Concerta, Ritalin). Based on the total number of prescriptions dispensed in the United States, there was a 463% increase (11.7 million) in amphetamine prescriptions from 1998 to 2007.[27] The number of methylphenidate prescriptions had remained relatively stable since 1996.[9]

Abuse Trend

Illicit use of prescription stimulants started to rise in the late 1990s, when there was a dramatic increase of prescriptions.[42] For example, the number of methylphenidate prescriptions had increased fivefold from 1991 to 1999.[42] In 2010, there were an estimated 1.1 million nonmedical users of stimulants, of which approximately 0.6 million were new users (see **Fig. 2**).[1] Unfortunately, the survey did not clearly state the number of users of different stimulants. Misuse of these drugs is common in adolescents and young adults. The mean age at which misuse of these drugs was initiated was 21.2 years old.[1] Prevalence of misuse were slightly higher among college-age students than high school students.[43] Approximately 10% to 12% of students in college or professional schools misused stimulants,[44,45] and approximately 31% of college students who were prescribed ADHD medications misused them.[46] According to Monitoring the Future study (a nationwide study conducted annually to monitor substance use in American Youth), prevalence rates of misuse were higher in high school students (approximately 8%) as compared to junior high school students (approximately 3%) in 2011.[47] The abuse trend for Ritalin in grades 8, 10, and 12 students showed an approximately 50% decrease in the past 10 years.[47] Caucasians, members of fraternities and sororities, individuals who partied more frequently, alcohol/marijuana users, and individuals with lower grade point averages were more likely to misuse stimulants.[43,44,48–51]

Compared to opioids or benzodiazepines, the number of ED visits related to prescription stimulants was low. In 2009, there were approximately 21,700 visits related to stimulants, with approximately 8700 involving amphetamine/dextroamphetamine and approximately 5000 involving methylphenidate (**Fig. 4**).[4] However, this represents a 276% increase in visits related to amphetamine/dextroamphetamine and a 102% increase in visits related to methylphenidate when compared to 2004 (see **Fig. 4**).[4] This shows an alarming increase of misuse of these drugs.

Misuse Motive

Most adolescents and young adults use stimulants to help them focus and study.[43,46,48] Others do so to get "high" or to experiment.[43,48] Prescription stimulants

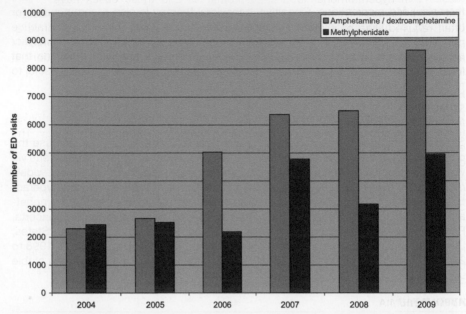

Fig. 4. ED visits related to stimulants. (*From* Substance Abuse and Mental Health Services Administration. Drug Abuse Warning Network, 2009: National estimates of drug-related emergency department visits. HHS Publication No. (SMA) 11-4659, DAWN Series D-35. Rockville (MD): Substance Abuse and Mental Health Services Administration, 2011.)

are perceived to be relatively safe considering they are prescribed to children.[42] They are also considered to be "better" than illicit drug like cocaine.[42] Most illicit users took the drugs orally, but some reported intranasal use.[46,48,51]

The increase of ADHD prescriptions has also increased the availability and accessibility of these drugs. The lifetime diversion rates with stimulant prescriptions were 16% to 29% among students.[43,46] Most abusers obtained their drug from friends with prescriptions.[47,51]

Adverse Effects

Usage of stimulants can cause headache, palpitations, hypertension, arrhythmias, depression, agitation and aggressiveness.[41,52] Abuse of these drugs can lead to tolerance and dependence, resulting in addiction, much like what cocaine and D-amphetamine (speed) do.[52] Severe overdose can result in convulsions, hallucinations, respiratory failure, or cardiac arrest.[41] Stimulants are known to increase heart rate and blood pressure, and have been associated with sudden death.[53] Although Canada Health has suspended the sales of Adderall XR in 2005, the FDA has not changed their recommendation on the use of these medications in the United States. In 2011, two large studies showed that ADHD medications (methylphenidate, amphetamine/dextroamphetamine, and others) did not increase risk of adverse cardiovascular events.[54,55] Based on these data, the FDA found that these drugs remain suitable for ADHD treatment, but warn that they should not be used in patients who have serious heart or blood pressure problems. In addition, the risk of adverse cardiovascular events remains for people who take large doses of the drugs in the abuse setting.

Preventive Measures

Considering that the most common motives for students to abuse stimulants is to help them focus and study, campaigns and programs aimed at educating students on healthy study habits and risks of prescription stimulants may help prevent misuse.[52] In addition, it is important for school and college administrators to be vigilant and hold students accountable for abusing stimulants. Substance abuse incidents should be documented, with issues followed up and addressed.[52] Health professionals need to properly counsel these young patients, and warn them of the danger of misuse as well as the legal ramifications of diverting drugs to others. Urine toxicology screens can be used to check for drug compliance. However, some of the ADHD medications such as Ritalin may not be screened easily in most laboratories owing to technological limitations. Testing is usually available on request as send-out to reference laboratories if needed.

SUMMARY

Although this review focuses on the abuse of prescription drugs in the United States, similar problems exist in Canada, Australia, the United Kingdom and other European countries.[34,55–59] Physicians face the difficult task of discerning drug-seekers from legitimate medical users. Practical guidelines on how to screen for drug-seeking patients are needed to help physicians from being fooled by abusers. Providers who overprescribe fuel the abuse epidemic and pose dangers to abusers. They could also face legal and licensing sanctions, particularly if they knowingly prescribe to drug seekers for illegal purposes. On the other hand, medical communities are often being criticized for not providing adequate care for conditions such as pain or anxiety, thus creating an unfortunate paradox.

Many of the prevention measures mentioned can be used to address misuse of different prescription drugs. For example, prescription drug monitoring programs are used to monitor the distribution and prescription pattern of controlled substances including opioids, benzodiazepines, barbiturates, and stimulants. They have been shown to help reduce "pharmacy/doctor shopping" and inappropriate prescriptions.[60] Similarly, the DEA monitors, investigates, and cracks down on all drug diversion cases (eg, pill mills). In addition, all businesses, pharmacies, and physicians must be registered with the DEA in order to manufacture, distribute, dispense, or prescribe controlled substances. The DEA also sets quotas to limit the manufacture and procurement of controlled substances. The goal is to put a ceiling on the production to limit drug diversion. However, this could also backfire. The DEA was recently being blamed for setting a quota too low for the manufacturers to produce enough Adderall to meet the demand, creating a drug shortage.[61]

The Office of National Drug Control Policy[62] under the Obama Administration also plays a key role in enhancing public awareness of prescription abuse and preventing drug abuse through various campaigns and programs. It works with other agencies to reduce abuse by supporting treatment and recovery efforts. In addition, it partners with other countries to reduce drug trafficking.

Other private companies such as Google, Bing, and Yahoo have adopted new policies to restrict online pharmacy advertising in 2010 to reduce the number of illegal online pharmacies. Under this policy, only pharmacies that are "Verified Internet Pharmacy Sites" that are certified by the National Association of Boards of Pharmacy and are in compliance with the pharmacy laws and practice standards in the United States can advertise on the sidebars of these Internet search engines.[3]

The abuse of prescription drugs is no doubt one of the fastest growing drug problems in the United States and is now being referred to as "epidemic" or "crisis."[24] The responsibilities to combat this problem reside not only with medical communities, governments, and law enforcement agencies, but also in the patients, parents, friends, and teachers. After all, most abusers obtained their supply of prescription drugs from people who had legitimate prescriptions.[1] It is imperative that everyone uses the prescriptions as indicated and not divert medications to others. Friends and families also need to be educated on the dangers of misuse. Everyone is responsible for cultivating an environment that promotes public health and safety. With the renewed effort to combat this epidemic, the hope is that the United States will become a healthier country.

REFERENCES

1. Substance Abuse and Mental Health Services Administration. Results from the 2010 National Survey on Drug Use and Health: summary of national findings, NSDUH Series H-41, HHS Publication No. (SMA) 11-4658. Rockville (MD): Substance Abuse and Mental Health Services Administration; 2011.
2. Warner M, Chen LH, Makuc DM, et al. Drug poisoning deaths in the United States, 1980–2008. NCHS Data Brief, 2011. Available at: www.cdc.gov.
3. U.S. Department of Justice National Drug Intelligence Center: National Drug Treat Assessment 2011. Product No. 2011-Q0317-001. Available at: http://www.justice.gov/archive/ndic/pubs44/44849/44849p.pdf. Accessed August 7, 2012.
4. Substance Abuse and Mental Health Services Administration. Drug Abuse Warning Network, 2009: National estimates of drug-related emergency department visits. HHS Publication No. (SMA) 11-4659, DAWN Series D-35. Rockville (MD): Substance Abuse and Mental Health Services Administration, 2011.
5. Bissell MG, Peat MA. Opioids 1: opiates. In: Magnani B, Bissell MG, Kwong TC, et al, editors. Clinical toxicology testing: a guide for laboratory professionals. Northfield (IL): CAP Press; 2012. p. 140–8.
6. Yu HE. Opioids 2: synthetic opioids. In: Magnani B, Bissell MG, Kwong TC, et al, editors. Clinical toxicology testing: a guide for laboratory professionals. Northfield (IL): CAP Press; 2012. p. 149–56.
7. Ingall GB, Vennapusa B. Opioids 3: synthetic opioids continued (methadone and buprenorphine). In: Magnani B, Bissell MG, Kwong TC, et al, editors. Clinical toxicology testing: a guide for laboratory professionals. Northfield (IL): CAP Press; 2012. p. 157–63.
8. Manchikanti L, Fellows B, Ailinani H, et al. Therapeutic use, abuse, and nonmedical use of opioids: a ten-year perspective. Pain Physician 2010;13(5):401–35.
9. National Institute on Drug Abuse. Research Report Series. Prescription drugs: abuse and addiction. NIH Publication No. 11-4881; 2011.
10. CDC Vital Signs Issue: Prescription Painkiller Overdoses in the US. November 2011. Available at: http://www.cdc.gov/vitalsigns. Accessed March 6, 2012.
11. Webster LR, Cochella S, Dasgupta N, et al. An analysis of the root causes for opioid-related overdose deaths in the United States. Pain Med 2011;12(Suppl 2): S26–35.
12. Paulozzi LJ, Kilbourne EM, Shah NG, et al. A history of being prescribed controlled substances and risk of drug overdose death. Pain Med 2012;13(1): 87–95.

13. Inciardi JA, Surratt HL, Cicero TJ, et al. Prescription opioid abuse and diversion in an urban community: the results of an ultrarapid assessment. Pain Med 2009; 10(3):537–48.

14. "Crime Inc" by CNBC Episode name: "Deadly Prescriptions". Available at: http://www.cnbc.com/id/42763325/. Accessed August 7, 2012.

15. Alam A, Gomes T, Zheng H, et al. Long-term analgesic use after low-risk surgery: a retrospective cohort study. Arch Intern Med 2012;172(5):425–30.

16. Strain EC. Assessment and treatment of comorbid psychiatric disorders in opioid-dependent patients. Clin J Pain 2002;18(4 Suppl):S14–27.

17. Joranson DE, Gilson AM. Drug crime is a source of abused pain medications in the United States. J Pain Symptom Manage 2005;30(4):299–301.

18. Greene D. Total necrosis of the intranasal structures and soft palate as a result of nasal inhalation of crushed OxyContin. Ear Nose Throat J 2005;84(8):512, 514, 516.

19. Rosenbaum CD, Boyle KL, Boyer EW. Nasopharyngeal necrosis after chronic opioid (oxycodone/acetaminophen) insufflation. J Med Toxicol 2012;8(2):240–1.

20. Jamison RN, Serraillier J, Michna D. Assessment and treatment of abuse risk in opioid prescribing for chronic pain. Pain Res Treat 2011;2011:941808.

21. Community-based opioid overdose prevention programs providing naloxone – United States, 2010. MMWR Morb Mortal Wkly Rep 2012;61:101–5.

22. Prescription Monitoring Programs Status. Available at: http://www.pmpalliance.org. Accessed June 20, 2012.

23. Centers for Disease Control and Prevention (CDC). CDC grand rounds: prescription drug overdoses-a U.S. epidemic. MMWR Morb Mortal Wkly Rep 2012;61(1):10–3.

24. Epidemic: responding to America's prescription drug abuse crisis. Available at: http://www.whitehouse.gov/sites/default/files/ondcp/issues-content/prescription-drugs/rx_abuse_plan.pdf. Accessed March 23, 2012.

25. "Massachusetts Blue Cross Blue Shield Initiates Pre-authorization for Painkillers to Control Drug Abuse." DARK Daily. Available at: http://www.darkdaily.com/massachusetts-blue-cross-blue-shield-initiates-pre-authorization-for-painkillers-to-control-drug-abuse-7-9-12#axzz22rczAULI. Accessed August 7, 2012.

26. Snyder ML, Melanson SE. Barbiturates. In: Magnani B, Bissell MG, Kwong TC, et al, editors. Clinical toxicology testing: a guide for laboratory professionals. Northfiled (IL): CAP Press; 2012. p. 126–31.

27. Belouin SJ, Reuter N, Borders-Hemphill V, et al. Prescribing trends for opioids, benzodiazepines, amphetamines, and barbiturates from 1998–2007. Available at: http://nac.samhsa.gov/DTAB/Presentations/Aug08/SeanBelouinDTAB0808_508.pdf. Accessed March 29, 2012.

28. Snyder ML, Melanson SE. Benzodiazepines. In: Magnani B, Bissell MG, Kwong TC, et al, editors. Clinical toxicology testing: a guide for laboratory professionals. Northfield (IL): CAP Press; 2012. p. 132–9.

29. Nutt DJ, Stahl SM, Searching for perfect sleep: the continuing evolution of GABAA receptor modulators as hypnotics. J Psychopharmacol 2010;24(11):1601–12.

30. Prescription sleep aid use in young adults. Available at: http://thomsonreuters.com/content/news_ideas/white_papers/healthcare/markupfielditems/Thomson_Reuters_Research_Br3.pdf. Accessed April 2, 2012.

31. Longo LP, Johnson B. Addiction: Part I. Benzodiazepines—side effects, abuse risk and alternatives. Am Fam Physician 2000;61(7):2121–8.

32. Kalapatapu, RK, Sullivan MA. Prescription use disorders in older adults. Am J Addict 2010;19(6):515–22.

33. Lader M. Benzodiazepines revisited—will we ever learn? Addiction 2011;106(12): 2086–109.

34. Lalive AL, Rudolph U, Luscher C, et al. Is there a way to curb benzodiazepine addiction? Swiss Med Wkly 2011;141:w13277.
35. Available at: http://www.justice.gov/dea. Accessed April 20, 2012.
36. Bronstein AC, Spyker DA, Cantilena LR Jr, et al. 2010 annual report of the American Association of Poison Control Centers' National Poison Data System (NPDS): 28th Annual Report. Clin Toxicol (Phila) 2011;49(10):910–41.
37. Work Group on Panic Disorder. American Psychiatric Association.Practice guideline for the treatment of patients with panic disorder. Am J Psychiatry 1998;155(5 Suppl):1–34.
38. el-Guebaly N, Sareen J, Stein MB. Are there guidelines for the responsible prescription of benzodiazepines? Can J Psychiatry 2010;55(11):709–14.
39. Morgenthaler T, Kramer M, Alessi C, et al. Practice parameters for the psychological and behavioral treatment of insomnia: an update. An American Academy of Sleep Medicine report. Sleep 2006;29(11):1415–9.
40. Sim MG, Khong E, Wain TD. The prescribing dilemma of benzodiazepines. Aust Fam Physician 2007;36(11):923–6.
41. Snyder ML, Melanson SE. Amphetamines. In: Magnani B, Bissell MG, Kwong TC, et al, editors. Clinical toxicology testing: a guide for laboratory professionals. Northfield (IL): CAP Press; 2012. p. 119–25.
42. Bogle KE, Smith BH. Illicit methylphenidate use: a review of prevalence, availability, pharmacology, and consequences. Curr Drug Abuse Rev 2009;2(2): 157–76.
43. Wilens TE, Adler LA, Adams J, et al. Misuse and diversion of stimulants prescribed for ADHD: a systematic review of the literature. J Am Acad Child Adolesc Psychiatry 2008;47(1):21–31.
44. Herman L, Shtayermman O, Aksnes B, et al. The use of prescription stimulants to enhance academic performance among college students in health care programs. J Physician Assist Educ 2011;22(4):15–22.
45. McNiel AD, Muzzin KB, DeWald JP, et al. The nonmedical use of prescription stimulants among dental and dental hygiene students. J Dent Educ 2011;75(3):365–76.
46. Rabiner DL, Anastopoulos AD, Costello EJ, et al. The misuse and diversion of prescribed ADHD medications by college students. J Atten Disord 2009;13(2):144–53.
47. The Monitoring the Future study: 2011 National results on adolescent drug use. Available at: http://monitoringthefuture.org/. Accessed March 5, 2012.
48. Teter CJ, McCabe SE, LaGrange K, et al. Illicit use of specific prescription stimulants among college students: prevalence, motives, and routes of administration. Pharmacotherapy 2006;26(10):1501–10.
49. Rabiner DL, Anastopoulos AD, Costello EJ, et al. Predictors of nonmedical ADHD medication use by college students. J Atten Disord 2010;13(6):640–8.
50. Arria AM, Wish ED. Nonmedical use of prescription stimulants among students. Pediatr Ann 2006;35(8):565–71.
51. Garnier-Dykstra LM, Caldeira KM, Vincent KB, et al. Nonmedical use of prescription stimulants during college: four-year trends in exposure opportunity, use, motives, and sources. J Am Coll Health 2012;60(3):226–34.
52. Rosenfield D, Hébert PC, Stanbrook MB, et al. Time to address stimulant abuse on our campuses. CMAJ 2011;183(12):1345.
53. Gould MS, Walsh BT, Munfakh JL, et al. Sudden death and use of stimulant medications in youths. Am J Psychiatry 2009;166(9):992–1001.
54. Cooper WO, Habel LA, Sox CM, et al. ADHD drugs and serious cardiovascular events in children and young adults. N Engl J Med 2011;365(20):1896–904.
55. Habel LA, Cooper WO, Sox CM, et al. ADHD medications and risk of serious cardiovascular events in young and middle-aged adults. JAMA 2011;306(24):2673–83.

56. Monheit B. Prescription drug misuse. Aust Fam Physician 2010;39(8):540–6.
57. Shield KD, Ialomiteanu A, Fischer B, et al. Non-medical use of prescription opioids among Ontario adults: data from the 2008/2009 CAMH Monitor. Can J Public Health 2011;102(5):330–5.
58. Bell J. The global diversion of pharmaceutical drugs: opiate treatment and the diversion of pharmaceutical opiates: a clinician's perspective. Addiction 2010;105(9): 1531–7.
59. Zacny JP, Lichtor SA. Nonmedical use of prescription opioids: motive and ubiquity issues. J Pain 2008;9(6):473–86.
60. Fisher J, Sanyal C, Frail D, et al. The intended and unintended consequences of benzodiazepine monitoring programmes: a review of the literature. J Clin Pharm Ther 2012;37(1):7–21.
61. "Adderall Drug Shortage Will Continue in 2012, Government Officials Say". ABC News, January 3, 2012. Available at http://abcnews.go.com/blogs/health/2012/01/03/adderall-drug-shortage-will-continue-in-2012-government-officials-say/. Accessed June 21, 2012.
62. Available at: http://www.whitehouse.gov/ondcp/. Accessed April 21, 2012.

Urine Drug Testing for Pain Management

Barbarajean Magnani, PhD, MD[a],*, Tai Kwong, PhD, DABCC[b]

KEYWORDS

- Opioids • Pain management • Drug compliance • Urine drug testing

KEY POINTS

- Opioid use is increasing producing an epidemic of unintentional drug poisoning deaths.
- Clinical guidelines for managing patients on chronic opioid (noncancer) pain therapy have been developed.
- There has been an increase in drug testing associated with chronic pain therapy and laboratories have been asked to assist in identifying compliant patients.
- Proper interpretation of positive/negative opiate results must take into consideration the metabolic pathways of opiates and assay limitations.
- Laboratorians are ready to help with testing strategies and interpretation of results.

INTRODUCTION

There is an epidemic of prescription drug abuse in the United States, which has created an increased burden on clinical toxicology laboratories and those who oversee drug testing. According to the 2009 report of the Drug Abuse Warning Network (DAWN), there were approximately 4.5 million drug-related visits to the emergency department, and the report revealed that more than 50% of the visits involved the nonmedical use of pharmaceuticals.[1] In this report, the nonmedical use of pharmaceuticals included (1) taking more than the prescribed dose of a prescription pharmaceutical, (2) taking more than the recommended dose of an over-the-counter pharmaceutical or supplement, (3) taking a pharmaceutical prescribed for another individual, (4) deliberate poisoning with a pharmaceutical by another person, and (5) documented misuse or abuse of a prescription drug, an over-the-counter pharmaceutical, or a dietary supplement.

Further scrutiny of the DAWN data revealed that almost 39% of the nonmedical use of pharmaceuticals involved opioids and 29% involved benzodiazepines (**Fig. 1**).

The authors have nothing to disclose.

[a] Department of Pathology and Laboratory Medicine, Tufts Medical Center, 800 Washington Street, Box 115, Boston MA 02115, USA; [b] Department of Pathology and Laboratory Medicine, University of Rochester, 601 Elmwood Avenue, Box 608, Rochester, NY 14642, USA
* Corresponding author.
E-mail address: bjmagnani@tuftsmedicalcenter.org

Clin Lab Med 32 (2012) 379–390
http://dx.doi.org/10.1016/j.cll.2012.07.001
0272-2712/12/$ – see front matter © 2012 Elsevier Inc. All rights reserved.

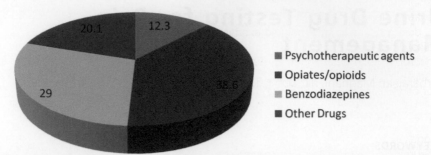

Fig. 1. Nonmedical use of pharmaceuticals. DAWN 2009. Percentage ED visits involving nonmedical use of pharmaceuticals. (*From* U.S. Department of Health and Human Services, Substance Abuse and Mental Health Services Administration, Center for Behavioral Health Statistics and Quality. The DAWN Report: highlights of the 2009 Drug Abuse Warning Network [DAWN] findings on drug-related emergency department visits. Rockville [MD]: Substance Abuse and Mental Health Services Administration; 2010. Available at: http://oas.samhsa.gov/2k10/dawn034/edhighlights.htm. Accessed June 15, 2012.)

Between 2004 and 2009 there was a particularly dramatic change in nonmedical use of opioids, with an increase to approximately 141%, and a 118% increase in the nonmedical use of benzodiazepines (**Fig. 2**).[1]

As a result of this increase in nonmedical use of prescription drugs there has been a concomitant rise in unintentional drug overdose deaths. In the early 1970s there were approximately 2 deaths per hundred thousand population and by 2007 the number was approaching almost 10 deaths per hundred thousand.[2] It is not surprising that there is such an increase in prescription drug–related deaths given that

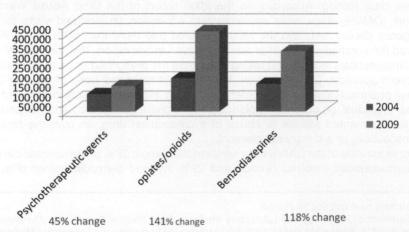

Fig. 2. Nonmedical use of pharmaceutical (ED visits DAWN 2009) Percent change from 2004 to 2009. (*From* U.S. Department of Health and Human Services, Substance Abuse and Mental Health Services Administration, Center for Behavioral Health Statistics and Quality. The DAWN Report: highlights of the 2009 Drug Abuse Warning Network [DAWN] findings on drug-related emergency department visits. Rockville [MD]: Substance Abuse and Mental Health Services Administration; 2010. Available at: http://oas.samhsa.gov/2k10/dawn034/edhighlights.htm. Accessed June 15, 2012.)

> **Box 1**
> **Clinical guidelines for opioid therapy for noncancer chronic pain**
>
> - Management of Opioid Therapy for Chronic Pain 2010. VA/DoD Clinical Practice Guidelines. United States Department of Veterans Affairs. Available at: http://www.healthquality.va.gov/Chronic_Opioid_Therapy_COT.asp. Accessed July 30, 2012.
>
> - Canadian Guideline for Safe and Effective Use of Opioids for Chronic Non-Cancer Pain, Parts A and B, 2010. National Opioid Use Guideline Group, Canada. Available at: http://nationalpaincentre.mcmaster.ca/opioid/. Accessed July 30, 2012.
>
> - Interagency Guideline on Opioid Dosing for Chronic Non-cancer Pain: An Educational Aid to Improve Care and Safety with Opioid Therapy, 2010 Update. Washington State Agency Medical Directors' Group. Available at: http://www.agencymeddirectors.wa.gov/Files/OpioidGdline.pdf. Accessed July 30, 2012.
>
> - Utah Clinical Guidelines on Prescribing Opioids for Treatment of Pain, 2009. Utah Department of Health. Available at: http://health.utah.gov/prescription/guidelines.html. Accessed July 30, 2012.
>
> - Clinical Guidelines for the Use of Chronic Opioid Therapy in Chronic Noncancer Pain, 2009. American Pain Society -American Academy of Pain Medicine Opioids Guidelines Panel. Available at: http://www.jpain.org/article/S1526-5900(08)00831-6/abstract. Accessed July 30, 2012.
>
> - Opioids in the Management of Chronic Non-Cancer Pain: An Update of American Society of the Interventional Pain Physicians' Guidelines, 2008. American Society of Interventional Pain Physicians. Available at: http://www.painphysicianjournal.com/2008/april/2008;11;S5-S62.pdf. Accessed July 30, 2012.

in the United States there are approximately 50 million people who experience chronic pain and 25 million who experience acute pain.[3] Pain is assessed as the fifth vital sign, and clinicians are obliged to address this problem. One hundred billion dollars is spent per year for pain care, and yet the economic loss due to a compromised workforce is approximately $60 billion per year.[3]

THE RESPONSE TO THE EPIDEMIC

In response to this epidemic, the White House Office of National Drug Control Policy created a Drug Abuse Prevention Plan in April of 2011.[4] This was a multiagency plan to stem the tide of prescription drug abuse. There are four key elements to the plan: (1) an expansion of the prescription drug monitoring programs (PDMP), (2) the responsible disposal of unused medications, (3) the reduction of pill mills through law enforcement efforts, and (4) support for education for both providers and patients. With respect to the last element, several state medical boards now require physicians to obtain continuing education credit in pain management and prescription opioid use (eg, California and Massachusetts).

Moreover, clinical practice guidelines have been published by state agencies and professional organizations with recommendations for safe practice of opioids therapy (see the list of guidelines in **Box 1**). These guidelines include a comprehensive initial evaluation of the patient with an assessment of the benefits and risks for opioid therapy. A thorough history and physical examination is warranted to determine the cause of pain, as well as a review of the psychosocial and family history factors, which may predict aberrant drug behavior. Factors that predict aberrant drug behavior include a personal or family history of alcohol or drug abuse, age between 16 and 45, preadolescent sexual abuse, and a history of psychological disorders including depression, attention deficit disorder, schizophrenia, bipolar disorder, and obsessive-compulsive disorder.[5,6] Tools for the clinician to aid in this assessment include standardized addiction screens (mental health and behavioral).

Additional guidelines emphasize the doctor-patient relationship and the importance of contracts or agreements. Patients need to have informed consent to understand potential risk factors associated with long-term opioid use, such as drowsiness, constipation, respiratory depression, and a potential for addiction. Clinicians should inform their patients of nonopioid alternatives to pain control and discuss treatment goals and therapeutic expectations, patient and clinician responsibilities, and indications for tapering or discontinuation of the medication such as adverse side effects and lack of therapeutic response.

Along with a consent form, there should be a medical agreement that stipulates the conditions and treatment plan with the long-term use of opioids. Although this is not a complete list, the treatment agreement plan should include the following: all controlled substances should come from the prescribing physician and be obtained from the same pharmacy where possible; the patient should inform the practitioner of any new medications, medical conditions, or adverse effects; the patient should not share or otherwise permit others to have access to these drugs; refills are contingent on keeping scheduled appointments; and unannounced urine or serum toxicology screens may be requested. The presence of unauthorized substances may prompt referral for assessment for addictive disorder.[6]

Last, the clinical guidelines require that patients be assessed periodically or with changing circumstances to see how they progress toward their therapeutic goal, that patients adhere to the prescribed therapies, and that adverse events, such as substance abuse or psychological issues, be addressed. Tools that the clinician can use to accomplish these goals include pill counts, family or caretaker interviews, prescription monitoring program data, and urine drug tests.

THE ROLE OF URINE DRUG TESTS IN CHRONIC OPIOID THERAPY

Urine drug tests provide objective evidence. Testing supplements self-reporting and behavioral monitoring and identifies problems that may otherwise go undetected such as the use of undisclosed medications, the nonuse of prescribed medications, or the use of alcohol and/or illicit drugs. The urine drug test is used extensively in attempts to document aberrant drug behavior and check for compliance to a prescribed medication(s).

Studies have shown that there is a high incidence of clinically unexpected urine drug test results among chronic pain patients being treated with opioids. In a retrospective study of 470 pain clinic patients in which urine drug testing results were reviewed and verified versus patients' medication histories by medical chart reviews, only 55% showed the appropriate opioid results (positive or negative), 10.3% were missing the prescribed opioid, 14.5% had an additional opioid, and 20.2% had an illicit substance.[7] In another study that looked at over 900,000 urines from chronic opioid patients, initially screened by immunoassay and if positive confirmed by tandem mass spectrometry, 11% had illicit drugs, 29% had nonprescribed drugs, and 38% had no prescribed drugs.[8]

THE TESTING MENU

A laboratory that provides drug testing service in support of pain management needs to be able to analyze a large number of different drugs. In one study of almost 14,000 pain clinic urine specimens being tested for opiates and other medications and illicit

| Box 2 |
| Synthetic opioids |

Buprenorphine

  Buprenex

  Subutex

  Suboxone

  Butran

Hydrocodone

  Hycodan

  Vicodin

Methadone

  Dolophine

Fentanyl

  Duragesic

Oxycodone

  OxyContin

  Percodan

  Oxecta

Hydromorphone

  Dilaudid

Tramadol

  Ultram

Tapentadol

  Nucynta

drugs, 22% of the specimens tested negative for opiates and 78% tested positive by immunoassays and were confirmed by gas chromatography/mass spectrometry (GC-MS). Of those, 63% had one drug confirmed, 26% had two drugs confirmed, and 11% had three or more drugs confirmed.[9] Drugs that should be considered when monitoring chronic noncancer pain patients include morphine, oxycodone, oxymorphone, hydrocodone, hydromorphone, dihydrocodeine, methadone, meperidine, fentanyl, and buprenorphine. A list of synthetic opioids can be found in **Box 2**. Typical illicit drugs should include amphetamines, benzodiazepines (although these may be prescribed therapeutically), cannabinoids, and cocaine.

DRUG TESTING ASSAYS

The initial test of a urine drug screen may be a panel of immunoassays, because most hospitals do not have the more sophisticated instrumentation such as GC-MS or tandem mass spectrometry (LC-MS/MS). Immunoassays are divided into two types of assays: class assays and analyte specific assays. Class assays include amphetamines, barbiturates, benzodiazepines, and opiates, whereas analyte-specific assays include cocaine (metabolite), cannabinoids, methadone (or metabolites), oxycodone,

Table 1 Opiates (ng/mL) giving positive opiates assay at 300 ng/mL cutoff						
	Opiates Immunoassays					
Drug	A	B	C	D	E	F
Morphine	300	300	300	300	300	300
Codeine	180	200	300	180	224	204
Hydromorphone	557	900	500	4000	1425	498
Dihydrocodeine	283	600	300	450	510	291
Hydrocodone	190	1000	300	1700	1086	247
Oxycodone	2644	1700	20000	16000	>75000	2550
Oxymorphone	2000	Unreactive	40000	. . .	40000	>20000

Abbreviations: A, Abbott Architect; B, Beckman; C, Biosite Triage; D, Microgenics DRI; E, Roche Cobas C; F, Syva EMIT.
Modified from Krasowski MD, Pizon AF, Siam MG, et al. Using molecular similarity to highlight the challenges of routine immunoassay-based drug of abuse/toxicology screening in emergency medicine. BMC Emerg Med 2009;9:5. Available at: http://www.biomedcentral.com/1471-227X/9/5. Accessed July 30, 2012.

buprenorphine, and fentanyl. Confirmation of an immunoassay-positive result would require more specific and sensitive instrumentation such as GC-MS or LC-MS/MS. These instruments offer lower cutoff concentrations and specific identification of a drug that produces a positive result in a class assay.[10]

IMMUNOASSAY LIMITATIONS

Specific identification of a drug producing a positive result is not possible with those immunoassays that are class assays. For example, a positive opiates assay may be positive because of one or more drugs including morphine, codeine, "heroin," or even hydrocodone. It is not possible for the ordering clinician to know conclusively that the patient is taking MS-Contin (morphine sulphate) when in fact the patient may have been taking hydrocodone or another opioid in addition to MS-Contin. This problem is due to the inherent lack of analyte specificity of the class assays and can only be overcome with technically specific assays. (There may be immunoassay analyte–specific tests, but many cases will still require definitive testing with either GC-MS or LC-MS/MS).

Immunospecificity

Certain immunoassays may lack immunospecificity for some target drugs. The assay antibody may have varying reactivities with the different drugs belonging to the same class. Thus, those drugs with lower cross-reactivities may escape detection. For example, depending on the specific opiate immunoassay, some are more or less sensitive to the various semisynthetic opioids (eg, hydromorphone, hydrocodone, oxycodone). **Table 1** shows the cross-reactivities of various opiates with common commercial opiate immunoassays at the 300 ng/mL cutoff. For assay A, codeine has a higher cross-reactivity than the calibrator morphine and it will produce a positive result at the 300 ng/mL cutoff when the concentration is only 180 ng/mL.[11] However, a hydromorphone result is very vendor assay–specific: assay C requires 500 ng/mL, whereas assay D requires 4000 ng/mL. Therefore, assay C is eight times more sensitive to hydromorphone than assay D. Similarly, Assay A is nine times more sensitive than assay D. Hydrocodone has better cross-reactivity to the class opiates screen than other semisynthetics, but each vendor assay is distinctive. Most opiates immunoassays are nonreactive to oxycodone, except perhaps assay B, and there is at least a 40 to 50 times difference in the cross-reactivities among the different assays. Low doses of oxycodone will clearly be missed, hence the need for a specific oxycodone assay.

All opiate assays are insensitive to the synthetic opioids (eg, methadone, buprenorphine, fentanyl). Detection of these opioids requires assays that specifically target these drugs; commercial immunoassays are available for oxycodone, buprenorphine, fentanyl, and methadone and its metabolites.

The same issues arise with the benzodiazepine class immunoassays having varying cross-reactivities with popular drugs such as alprazolam and clonazepam.[12] Identification of the specific drug is not possible with immunoassays and, if needed, urines producing positive results will also require further testing. The clinical laboratory should understand the limitations of the immunoassays it offers and communicate the limitations to the end users.

Cutoff Concentrations

Other issues that arise with immunoassays are related to assay cutoff. This cutoff is the threshold concentration above which the test result is considered to be positive (drug present) and below which the result is considered to be negative, although a negative result does not equate to absence of drug. For example, if the threshold concentration for positive is 300 ng/mL and the result is 299 ng/mL, it is probable that the urine contained drug, but the concentration is insufficient to be reported as positive.

Some assays have flexibility within the manufacturer's specifications to choose one of several cutoff concentrations (eg, benzodiazepines) in order to tailor the assay to the users' specifications. One must balance the ability to detect certain drugs (triazolobenzodiazepines) with the lower cutoff without confounding the assay with false-positives, which may be picked up at lower cutoff concentrations. In addition, there are assays with different cutoffs that are distinct assays, such as the opiate assays, with cutoff concentrations at 2000 ng/mL and 300 ng/mL. For the hospital setting, the 300 ng/mL assay is appropriate and is better at detecting some of the semisynthetic opioids. The 2000 ng/mL assay is primarily useful in workplace drug testing where the aim of the assay is to detect heroin abuse, not drugs used specifically for pain management, and the higher cutoff is set to reduce positive opiate results due to consumption of contaminated poppy seeds.[13]

Other considerations include cross-reactivities with the specific opioid immunoassays such as oxycodone, methadone, and buprenorphine, for example. Minor nonspecificity can give a false-positive result and this will remain undetected unless confirmation is performed. Even a .01% cross-reactivity could produce a false-positive result if the interfering substance concentration is very high and the target analyte cutoff is low. For example 50,000 ng/mL of morphine with a .01% cross-reactivity gives an apparent buprenorphine concentration of 5 ng/mL, which is the cutoff for one frequently used buprenorphine assay.[14] As a result of potential cross-reactivity, some laboratories have raised their cutoff concentration for buprenorphine to 10, 20, 30, or even 50 ng/mL.

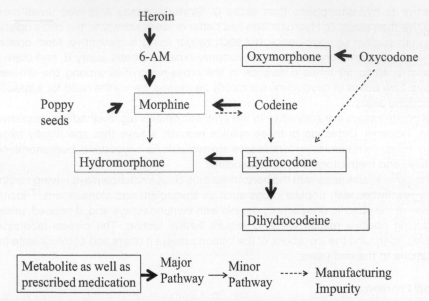

Fig. 3. Opiates' metabolic pathways. (*Courtesy* of Dr. Tai Kwong, PhD, DABCC.)

TANDEM MASS SPECTROMETRY

LC-MS/MS–based assays are analytically more sensitive and have cutoff concentrations based on limits of detection and quantitation that are lower than those used for immunoassays. This assay allows not only identification of specific drugs, but also detection at concentrations that are missed by the higher concentration cutoff used with immunoassays. For example, the opiates (morphine) immunoassay cutoff concentration is 300 ng/mL, whereas that used for LC-MS/MS is 50 ng/mL, a sixfold lower detection limit and therefore increased in detection rate. For those semisynthetic opioids that have lower cross-reactivities with the opiate immunoassay, such as hydromorphone and hydrocodone, the advantage gained by the lower LC-MS/MS cutoff is even more dramatic.[15]

Whereas the use of high sensitivity mass spectrometry assays includes specific identification of parent compounds and their metabolites, and the ability to detect low concentrations of analytes, there are disadvantages. These techniques are more costly and technically challenging, and the ability to detect very low concentrations of drugs may complicate the interpretation of results because both minor metabolites and pharmaceutical impurities may now be detected.

INTERPRETATION OF OPIATES RESULTS

Interpretation of opiates results can be challenging, both with immunoassay testing as well as with the more technically sophisticated assays. **Fig. 3** shows the opiates metabolic pathways, which includes the major pathways, minor pathways, and manufacturing impurities. A minor metabolite can also be a prescription opiate (eg, hydromorphone is a metabolite of morphine), and understanding the relative concentrations of the opiates present can help determine whether the unexpected opiate is a minor metabolite of the prescribed opiate or a nonprescribed opiate (**Table 2**). With a patient on MS-Contin the opiates immunoassay would be positive (at the 300 ng/mL

Table 2 Interpretation of drug test result: need for quantitation		
	Patient on MS Contin	
Opiate(s) Present (ng/mL)	Opiates IA Result[a]	Source of Morphine
Morphine 500	POS	Poppy seeds
Morphine 50,000	POS	MS Contin
Morphine 50,000 Hydromorphone 500	POS	MS Contin
Morphine 50,000 Hydromorphone 5,000	POS	MS Contin Dilaudid

Abbreviation: IA, immunoassay; POS, positive.
[a] 300 ng/mL cutoff.

cutoff), but a concentration of 500 ng/mL versus 50,000 ng/mL would have a very different interpretation. The lower concentration could be attributed to ingestion of poppy seeds that are contaminated with morphine (and a smaller amount of codeine),[16] whereas the higher concentration would be consistent with administration of prescription morphine. With LC-MS/MS, the additional findings of hydromorphone could be interpreted as being the minor pathway metabolite of morphine, or at higher concentrations, due to its use as an additional (not prescribed) drug (Dilaudid).[17] Another minor metabolite of codeine is hydrocodone (see **Fig. 3**).[18]

Low concentrations of opiates can be traced to impurities produced during pharmaceutical manufacturing processes: hydrocodone and codeine are impurities in pharmaceutical preparations of oxycodone and morphine, respectively.[19,20]

CLINICAL CONSIDERATIONS

The opportunity for the laboratory to provide assistance in the interpretation of results and in the ordering of the correct tests cannot be overemphasized. The challenges faced by clinicians in managing these patients are broad, and expertise offered by the laboratory is usually welcome. How proficient are nonlaboratory physicians in interpreting urine drug tests? In a seven multiple-choice survey administered to 150 physicians at an opioid education meeting, 68% had used drug tests with their patient population and 76% had prescribed opioids. Additionally, 19% were board certified in pain management and 6% in addiction medicine or psychiatry. Of those who ordered drug tests, none had seven correct answers and only 30% scored more than half correctly.[21] It is clear from these data that clarification on test result interpretation is a vital role the laboratory can play in caring for these patients.

Consider the following case: a 62-year-old man with postlaminectomy syndrome prescribed morphine sulfate and oxycodone (to be taken 15 mg twice a day and 30 mg twice a day, respectively) presents to the physician for an increase in pain medication to control worsening pain. The patient has a positive opiates immunoassay result. The clinician is reassured by the positive opiates screen but wants to know if this patient is taking the prescribed medications before he increases the dosage. The results of further analysis can be seen in **Table 3**. Although the patient has morphine present, there is no oxycodone or its metabolite oxymorphone present in the urine. This result would lead the clinician to conclude that the patient is noncompliant with respect to oxycodone and also consider the possibility of diversion and address this possibility prior to prescribing additional pain medication.

| Table 3 | |
| Opiates, expanded (LC-MS/MS; urine) | |
Test	Results
Codeine	Negative
Hydrocodone	Negative
Oxycodone	Negative
Morphine	2800 ng/ml
Hydromorphone	Negative
Oxymorphone	Negative

Another patient prescribed Percocet and MS-Contin for chronic joint pain is now under scrutiny by the prescribing rheumatologist because her urine screen tested positive for amphetamines by immunoassay. Testing by LC-MS/MS did not confirm these results, and further review of the patient's medication list revealed that she is also taking trazodone. It is known that a metabolite of trazodone, meta-chlorophenylpiperazine (m-CPP) can cross-react with the amphetamine assay and cause a false-positive enzyme immunoassay screen.[22] This is an important finding because many chronic pain opioids contracts may be considered in jeopardy if the patient is using illicit drugs while on opioid therapy.

A 60-year-old man with chronic leg pain is prescribed Percocet and Duragesic 75 by (fentanyl), and his urine drug screen is positive for the opiate immunoassay. The clinician wants to be sure that these results are consistent with his medications. The opiate immunoassay does not cross-react with fentanyl or its major metabolite, norfentanyl, and unless there are high concentrations of oxycodone/oxymorphone present, it is unlikely that these drugs would produce a positive opiate immunoassay result. On expansion of the opiates screen using LC-MS/MS to identify what opioids are producing the positive result, morphine at 430 ng/mL is detected (6-monoacetylmorphine, 6-AM, is not detected). How can this result be explained to the clinician? Several explanations can be offered: Given the negative oxycodone/oxymorphone and fentanyl results, it is clear that the patient is not taking any fentanyl or oxycodone/acetaminophen, which could place the chronic pain contract in jeopardy. It is also clear that the immunoassay screen was positive because of the presence of morphine. Where did the morphine come from? One consideration could be heroin abuse, although the lack of 6-AM and the low concentration of morphine do not support this conclusion (6-AM is an intermediate metabolite in the metabolism of diacetylmorphine or heroin), another could be the consumption of contaminated poppy seeds.[16] On further investigation of the medical record, it was noted that the patient had been treated in the emergency department the evening before and received morphine for pain intravenously. This fact was not known to the physician responsible for the patient's chronic pain treatment. Part of the patient contract is to inform the prescribing physician of any changes in the original plan and any additional treatments. Here is a case in which the laboratory was able to help sort out the meaning of the positive results and provide the clinician with a clearer picture of his patient.

SUMMARY

Drug testing as an adjunct to managing patients on chronic opioids is critical. It is an objective means to determine compliance (to some degree) with the program and can help identify drugs that should be in the patient's system, as well as those that should not be in the patient's system. Given the increase in prescription opioid use by the population and the complications of understanding the drug testing results, laboratorians will have an increased need in understanding the testing assays to provide the implications of the testing results.

REFERENCES

1. U.S.Department of Health and Human Services, Substance Abuse and Mental Health Services Administration, Center for Behavioral Health Statistics and Quality. The DAWN Report: highlights of the 2009 Drug Abuse Warning Network (DAWN) findings on drug-related emergency department visits. Rockville (MD): Substance Abuse and Mental Health Services Administration; 2010. Available at: http://oas.samhsa.gov/2k10/dawn034/edhighlights.htm. Accessed June 15, 2012.
2. National Vital Statistics System, Center for Disease Control and Prevention.
3. Trescot AM, Helm S, Hansen H, et al. Opioids in the management of chronic non-cancer pain: an update of American Society of the Interventional Pain Physicians' (ASIPP) Guidelines. Pain Physician 2008;11:S5–62.
4. White House Office of National Drug Control Policy. 2011 prescription drug abuse prevention plan. Available at: http://www.whitehouse.gov/ondcp/prescription-drug-abuse. Accessed June 15, 2012.
5. Hammett-Stabler CA, Webster L. Urine drug testing: augmenting pain management & enhancing patient care. PharmaCom Group, 2008.
6. Chou R, Fanciullo GJ, Fine PG, et al. Clinical guidelines for the use of chronic opioid therapy in chronic noncancer pain. J Pain 2009;10:113–30.
7. Michna E, Jamison RN, Loc-Duyen, et al. Urine toxicology screening among chronic pain patients on opioid therapy: frequency and predictability of abnormal findings. Clin J Pain 2007;23:173–9.
8. Couto J, Romney M, Leider H, et al. High rate of inappropriate drug use in the chronic pain population. Popul Health Manag 2009;12:185–90.
9. Cone EJ, Caplan YH, Black DL, et al. Urine drug testing of chronic pain patients: licit and illicit drug patterns. J Anal Toxicol 2008;32:530–43.
10. Hammett-Stabler C, Magnani BJ. Supporting the pain service. In: Magnani BJ, Bissell M, Kwong T. Clinical toxicology testing. Northfield (IL): CAP Press; 2012. p. 15–26.
11. Krasowski MD, Pizon AF, Siam MG, et al. Using molecular similarity to highlight the challenges of routine immunoassay-based drug of abuse/toxicology screening in emergency medicine. BMC Emerg Med 2009;9:5.
12. Snyder M, Melanson S. Benzodiazepines. In: Magnani BJ, Bissell M, Kwong T. Clinical toxicology testing. Northfield (IL): CAP Press; 2012. p. 132–9.
13. Federal Register. Notice changing the opiate testing cutoff concentrations [effective December 1, 1998]. Available at: http://dwp.samhsa.gov/DrugTesting/Files_Drug_Testing/Notices_Docs_Resources/FR_Final/Federal%20Register%20Notice%20Changing%20the%20Opiate%20Testing%20Cutoff%20Concentrations.html. Accessed June 23, 2012.
14. Bottcher M, Beck O. Evaluation of buprenorphine CEDIA assay versus GC-MS and ELISA using urine samples from patients in substitution treatment. J Anal Toxicol 2005;29:769–76.
15. Mikel C, Almazan P, West R, et al. LC-MS/MS extends the range of drug analysis in pain patients. Ther Drug Monit 2009;31:746–8.
16. ElSohly HN, ElSohly MA, Standford DF. Poppy seed ingestion of opiate urinalysis: a closer look. J Anal Toxicol 1990;14:308–10

17. Cone E, Caplan Y, Moser F, et al. Evidence that morphine is metabolized to hydromorphone but not to oxymorphone. J Anal Toxicol 2008;32:319–23.
18. Oyler J, Cone E, Joseph R, et al. Identification of hydrocodone in human urine following controlled codeine administration. J Anal 2000;24:530–5.
19. West R, West C, Crews B, et al. Anomalous observations of hydrocodone in patients on oxycodone. Clin Chim Acta 2011;412:29–32.
20. West R, Crews B, Mikel C, et al. Anomalous observations of codeine in patients on morphine. Ther Drug Monit 2009;31:776–8.
21. Reisfield G, Bertholf R, Barkin R, et al. Urine drug test interpretation: what do physicians know? J Opioid Management 2007;3:80–6.
22. Baron J, Griggs D, Nixon A, et al. The trazodone metabolite meta-chlorophenyl-peperazine can cause false-positive urine amphetamine immunoassay results. J Anal Toxicol 2011;35:363–8.

Alcohol Biomarkers

Glynnis B. Ingall, MD, PhD

KEYWORDS

- Carbohydrate-deficient transferrin • Acetaldehyde adducts
- Ethyl glucuronide • Ethyl sulfate • Phosphatidylethanol • Fatty acid ethyl esters

KEY POINTS

- Excessive alcohol consumption poses a wide variety of significant immediate and long-term health risks.
- Ethanol biomarkers have clinical utility for detection, diagnosis, and treatment of alcohol use disorders and for screening for fetal alcohol exposure.
- Indirect biomarkers are those that reflect the toxic effects of ethanol on organs, tissues, or body biochemistry, whereas direct biomarkers are products of ethanol metabolism.
- Indirect biomarkers include liver enzymes (aspartate aminotransferase, alanine aminotransferase, and γ-glutamyltransferase), carbohydrate-deficient transferrin, and mean corpuscular volume.
- Direct biomarkers include acetaldehyde adducts, ethyl glucuronide, ethyl sulfate, phosphatidylethanol, and the fatty acid ethyl esters.

INTRODUCTION

Excessive alcohol consumption poses significant immediate and long-term health risks. The search for sensitive and specific laboratory tests suitable for screening, diagnosis, and risk/severity assessment of patients with alcohol use disorders and for monitoring and motivating patients undergoing rehabilitation treatment for alcohol abuse is an active area of clinical research. The other growing use of these biomarkers is for maternal and neonatal screening. These markers can potentially be applied to the management of pregnant women with alcohol use disorders and may allow for earlier identification and treatment of infants at risk for fetal alcohol syndrome and related disorders. A number of promising alcohol biomarkers are being investigated for their potential applications in these settings. These biomarkers fall into two categories, indirect and direct. Indirect markers are those that reflect the toxic effects of ethanol on organs, tissues, or body biochemistry. Direct biomarkers are products

The author has nothing to disclose.
Department of Pathology, MSC08 4640, 1 University of New Mexico Health Sciences Center, Albuquerque, NM 87131, USA
E-mail address: gingall@salud.unm.edu

of ethanol metabolism. The most promising of these direct markers are the longer-lived, nonoxidative products of ethanol metabolism.[1-4]

EPIDEMIOLOGY OF ALCOHOL USE DISORDERS

A significant proportion of the U.S. population is current alcohol consumers, and some of these individuals use it to excess. The 2010 National Survey on Drug Use and Health found that about one half of the population (older than 12 years old) drinks alcohol. Furthermore, about one quarter of drinkers reported that they had experienced binge drinking and 6.7% were identified as heavy drinkers. Many youths aged 12 to 17 years also report that they use alcohol with rates for drinking of 13.7%, binge drinking, 7.8%; and heavy drinking, 1.7%. About 10% of pregnant women aged 15 to 44 years reported binge drinking during the first trimester of pregnancy.[5] U.S. Centers for Disease Control and Prevention (CDC) studies have indicated that from 0.2 to 1.5 cases of fetal alcohol syndrome (FAS) occur per 1000 births. Individuals exhibiting some but not all the diagnostic features of FAS are defined as having fetal alcohol spectrum disorders (FASD). It is estimated that there may be three times as many cases of FASD as FAS.[6]

The CDC has estimated that about 80,000 deaths annually in the United States are attributable to alcohol use disorders, which translates to 2.3 million years of potential life lost per year (2001–2005). In 2005, more than 1.6 million hospitalizations and at least 4 million emergency department (ED) visits were related to excessive alcohol consumption.[7]

PHYSIOLOGIC EFFECTS AND TOXICITY OF ETHANOL
Acute Consumption of Ethanol

The primary acute manifestation of ethanol consumption is central nervous system (CNS) depression. Ethanol affects many neurochemical processes, resulting in an imbalance of excitatory and inhibitory pathways. Signs of intoxication are seen in most individuals after two to three drinks. Initially the individual may show stimulatory effects and behavior related to loss of inhibitions. As the blood ethanol concentrations rise, the depressant effects predominate. Blood ethanol concentrations above 300 mg/dL may lead to coma and death. Other acute effects of ethanol are depression of central temperature regulatory functions, diuresis due to suppression of antidiuretic hormone, and acute pancreatitis and gastritis.[8]

Chronic Use of Ethanol

Chronic ethanol use has untoward effects on many organ systems. Brain disorders associated with chronic excessive ethanol consumption include alcoholic dementia and cognitive deficits, brain atrophy, Wernicke–Korsakoff syndrome and cerebellar degeneration, among others. Chronic heavy ethanol use increases the risk for a number of cardiovascular disorders including myocardial infarction, hypertension, cardiac arrhythmias, congestive heart failure, and hemorrhagic strokes. An alcohol use disorder should be considered as a possible causative factor in patients presenting with gastrointestinal complaints such as chronic gastritis and pancreatitis, esophageal disorders, chronic diarrhea, malabsorption, hepatitis, and hepatic cirrhosis. Alcoholics are also prone to nutritional disorders, macrocytic anemia, thrombocytopenia, and immune system depression.[8]

Tolerance and Dependence

Tolerance is defined as diminished psychological and physiologic response to the same dose. Ethanol is associated with both acute and chronic tolerance to its effects.

The tolerance that occurs after chronic exposure to ethanol is in part metabolic in nature due to enzyme induction.

Chronic heavy alcohol users may develop a physical dependence. These individuals exhibit a withdrawal syndrome when deprived of ethanol. Symptoms vary in severity depending on the duration and extent of ethanol consumption and may manifest as wakefulness, nausea, anxiety, hallucinations, delirium, tremors, tachycardia, and, in severe cases, seizures and death. Psychological dependence (craving and strong desire to obtain more ethanol) may also be exhibited.[8]

Teratogenic Effects

Fetal exposure to ethanol as a result of maternal consumption, especially during the first trimester of pregnancy, may result in fetal alcohol syndrome in the child. Features of this syndrome are characteristic cranial/facial abnormalities, CNS dysfunction (hyperactivity, attention deficit, mental retardation, and learning disabilities) and growth retardation.[8]

METABOLISM OF ETHANOL

Ethanol consumed orally is absorbed rapidly from the gastrointestinal tract (stomach and small intestine) into the blood. The major site of ethanol metabolism is the liver (90%–98%), with the remainder excreted in urine, sweat, and breath.

Oxidative Metabolism

Two oxidative enzymes mediate the predominate pathway of ethanol metabolism in the liver. Cytoplasmic alcohol dehydrogenase converts ethanol to acetaldehyde followed by mitochondrial aldehyde dehydrogenase, which converts acetaldehyde to acetic acid. These steps require NAD^+, which can become depleted during ethanol metabolism resulting in zero-order kinetics (constant amount metabolized per unit time). This reduction of NAD^+ availability alters the activities of other NAD^+-dependent enzymes leading to a variety of metabolic consequences such as lactate accumulation, reduced tricarboxylic acid (TCA) cycle activity, elevated acetyl coenzyme A, and increased fatty acid synthesis, among other effects.[8] The microsomal enzyme cytochrome P450 2E1 (CYP2E1) mediates another hepatic oxidative pathway. This cytochrome is inducible by chronic ethanol use. Induction not only increases acetaldehyde production from ethanol but can also enhance the metabolism of other (CYP2E1) substrates leading to toxin activation. By reducing the availability of NADPH and promoting the formation of reactive oxygen containing radicals, the metabolism of ethanol by CPY2E1 creates oxidative stress. This is believed to be one of the mechanisms of ethanol-induced cell injury or death.[8] Furthermore, the oxygen radicals can interact with lipids to form reactive molecules via lipid peroxidation. These molecules can bind covalently with proteins, forming adducts.[9] The acetaldehyde generated by ethanol oxidation is also known to form adducts with a variety of macromolecules. These adducts have been studied for their potential as alcohol biomarkers.

Nonoxidative Metabolism

Nonoxidative pathways account for only a small proportion of the overall metabolism of ethanol. Products of these pathways include ethyl glucuronide, ethyl sulfate, phosphatidylethanol (PEth), and fatty acid ethyl esters (FAEEs). Nevertheless, it is these relatively minor products of nonoxidative pathways that show the most promise as potential alcohol biomarkers.[1–3]

BIOMARKERS RELATED TO THE TOXIC EFFECTS OF ALCOHOL (INDIRECT MARKERS)

For many years, several readily available laboratory tests have been used clinically as indicators of heavy alcohol consumption. Included in this group of tests are aspartate aminotransferase (AST) and alanine aminotransferase (ALT), γ-glutamyltransferase (GGT), and mean corpuscular volume (MCV). A newer biomarker, carbohydrate-deficient transferrin (CDT, singly or in combination with GGT), is becoming a more frequently requested test to detect alcohol use disorders. These analytes are all considered indirect markers of ethanol exposure because they reflect the toxic effects of ethanol on tissues and biochemical pathways. In general, these tests have limited specificity, since these parameters may be abnormal due to other conditions and disease states in the absence of alcohol exposure.[1–3]

Liver Enzymes

GGT is a hepatic microsomal enzyme. Serum GGT may be increased due to release from liver cells damaged by alcohol, hepatotoxic drugs, ischemia, and viral hepatitis, among other causes.[2] Another cause of elevated GGT is induction by alcohol or other drugs such as barbiturates and phenytoin. Of the liver enzymes, GGT is the most sensitive marker for alcohol use.[3] It takes about 2 to 3 weeks for GGT to recover to baseline after cessation of alcohol use, making this marker less beneficial as a monitor for abstinence.[1,3] Furthermore, the clinical value of GGT as a screening test for ethanol use disorders is limited by false positives due to conditions such as nonalcoholic liver diseases, hepatobiliary disorders, obesity, diabetes, smoking, and induction of GGT synthesis by other medications. The overall sensitivity of GGT is moderate for detection of heavy ethanol use, and its effectiveness as a screen is variable depending on the population studied and the prevalence of alcohol use disorders and other non-alcohol–related factors that increase GGT.[3]

The transaminases ALT and AST have also been used as indicators of heavy alcohol use. ALT is found only in hepatocytes. AST is present in many different tissues but predominates in liver and skeletal muscle. Consequently, AST elevations are not necessarily specific to the liver. Both AST and ALT can be elevated as the result of hepatocellular damage. A ratio of AST to ALT greater than 2 suggests that the liver damage is more likely to be due to alcohol than to other causes. The transaminases are not as sensitive or specific for heavy alcohol use as GGT and CDT are.[1,3,10–12]

CDT

Transferrin is a glycoprotein synthesized in the liver. It functions as an iron transport protein. Transferrin has different isoforms that vary in the number of terminal sialic acid residues. CDT refers to isoforms that are deficient in sialic acid. CDT is usually defined as the disialo, monosialo, and asialo isoforms of transferrin. Heavy ethanol abuse increases the fraction of CDTs.[12,13]

CDT is readily available as a clinical diagnostic test for alcohol use disorders. This test has moderate sensitivity and specificity and is a longer-term marker of heavy ethanol use.[1] Consumption of 50 to 80 g alcohol per day for 1 to 2 weeks elevates CDT above baseline.[14] CDT is especially useful as a marker for abstinence because it has a relatively short half-life (1.5 weeks) and returns to baseline levels 2 to 5 weeks after ethanol cessation. Abstinence would be supported by the fact that CDT is declining even though other alcohol markers such as liver enzymes may still be elevated.[13,15]

There are a number of clinical and analytical factors to consider to optimize CDT assays and the resulting interpretation. Reported CDT values and reference intervals resulting from various methods are quite variable depending on the standards used and fractions measured. Most high-performance liquid chromatography (HPLC) and capillary electrophoresis (CE) methods report CDT as % DST (disialotransferrin fraction to total transferrin) or as the sum of asialotransferrin and disialotransferrin. Immunoassay methods differ in the fractions detected depending on reagent antibody reactivity and specificity. It is now recommended to report CDT as a percent of total transferrin so as to at least partially correct for the changes in transferrin production due to underlying physiologic states (iron deficiency or overload, pregnancy, female hormone status, among others).[16,17]

The advantage of HPLC and CE over immunoassay is that these methods allow for separation and quantification of individual isoforms and the detection of transferrin genetic variants and other interfering proteins that may affect analysis and interpretation of results. CE methods, however, may show interference by comigrating proteins because of the relatively nonspecific UV detectors on these instruments. Interference by hemoglobin–haptoglobin complexes may occur in HPLC methods that utilize absorption of the iron–transferrin complex at 460 to 470 nm for detection.[13,15]

Alterations in CDT levels are not entirely specific for alcohol use. Individuals with rare congenital disorders of glycosylation (carbohydrate-deficient glycoprotein syndrome) may have elevated CDT. Furthermore, patients with advanced chronic liver disease may have high CDT values in the absence of ethanol intake. Some studies continue to report more false positives in women even with the newer % CDT tests.[17,18] Overall, however, CDT appears to be a more specific alcohol marker with fewer false positives than the liver enzymes or MCV.

It should be noted that results of past clinical studies related to CDT as a marker of ethanol abuse are difficult to interpret because of conflicting findings. The reported variation in CDT test specificity and sensitivity for populations differing in gender, ethnicity, age, or body mass index (BMI) may be related, in part, to the analytical method used to measure CDT rather than to true differences in the populations studied.[19] The utility of this test should be enhanced by standardization and improvement in analytical methods and use of % CDT rather than CDT absolute values.[15]

MCV

MCV is a measure of red blood cell size and is a routine hematologic parameter. The average MCV is higher in heavy drinkers and there appears to be a positive correlation between extent of drinking and the size of the red blood cells.[20] In general, MCV does not appear to be as sensitive as either GGT or CDT for detection of alcohol use. MCV is not a suitable marker for abstinence because it may take 2 to 4 months to reach baseline levels after ethanol consumption has stopped.[11,20] MCV is limited as a screen for alcohol use because it is elevated by many other conditions such as vitamin B_{12} or folate deficiency, hypothyroidism, and hemolytic anemia, among others.

Indirect Marker Comparison and Combined Marker Panels

A number of clinical studies have been designed to compare the diagnostic value of the various indirect markers of alcohol when used singly or as multimarker panels. CDT and GGT appear to be independent markers for heavy drinking. Most studies have shown that both CDT and GGT are about equal in sensitivity for detection of heavy alcohol use. However, the specificity of CDT is higher.[14] CDT is less affected by medications and non-alcohol–related disease states. Therefore, it may be a better marker than GGT in the acute care setting, where it is common to have patients with underlying conditions or medications that increase their GGT levels. In outpatient clinics, improved sensitivity in screening for alcoholism may be achieved through combination of the two markers (CDT–GGT). As in any screening protocol, the positive predictive value of these tests would be influenced by the prevalence of heavy drinking in the population.[21]

In a study that evaluated % CDT, GGT, and MCV in alcohol-dependent individuals (currently using alcohol) to social drinkers, CDT was found to be most sensitive (73.3%), GGT slightly less sensitive (71.3%), and MCV least sensitive (64.4%.). The possibility that the sensitivity of % CDT could be improved if it were combined with other common laboratory tests (GGT, MCV, AST, ALT levels, among others) was further investigated. Using multivariate analysis, only the combination % CDT with GGT or MCV resulted in enhanced diagnostic efficiency.[22]

In another investigation, the combined GGT–CDT marker was compared to conventional alcohol markers. The sensitivity for detection of heavy drinkers was best for the combined GGT–CDT test (90%), followed by CDT (63%), GGT (58%), ALT (50%), AST (47%), and MCV (45%). Furthermore, the sensitivity of the combined GGT–CDT test was essentially the same in alcoholics with liver disease as in those without liver disease.[23]

BIOMARKERS DERIVED FROM ALCOHOL METABOLIC PRODUCTS (DIRECT MARKERS)

Minor products of ethanol metabolism have been evaluated for their clinical and forensic potential as alcohol biomarkers. The most promising of these markers are acetaldehyde adducts, ethyl glucuronide (EtG), ethyl sulfate (EtS), phosphatidylethanol (PEth), and fatty acid ethyl esters (FAEEs).

Acetaldehyde Adducts

Adducts formed through covalent binding of acetaldehyde to tissue and blood macromolecules (protein, DNA, and lipids) have been studied for many years. Furthermore, adducts related to ethanol-induced lipid peroxidation products are subjects of active ongoing research into the pathogenesis of alcohol-mediated diseases and alcohol-associated neoplasia. The binding of ethanol metabolic products to macromolecules causes deleterious effects through alteration of protein structure and functions or through mutagenic changes in DNA.[9,11,24,25] These adducts are also known to be immunogenic. Antibodies to acetaldehyde-modified proteins have been detected in alcohol abusers.[26] Such antibodies have been proposed as another potential alcohol biomarker.

Acetaldehyde hemoglobin has the greatest potential as an alcohol biomarker. However, testing for acetaldehyde hemoglobin is not readily available for practical clinical use at this time. The methods used to measure acetaldehyde adducts in biological specimens are immunoassay or HPLC techniques. Immunoassay development has been challenging due to difficulties in generating reproducible and specific reagent antibodies and selection of the most appropriate adducts as targets for reagent antibody production. Chromatographic methods require sensitivity to measure hemoglobin fractions that are less than 1% of total hemoglobin as well as good separation from the other hemoglobins present in whole blood specimens. Improved separation of acetaldehyde–hemoglobin from glycated hemoglobins has been reported through the use of cation-exchange HPLC. Using this method, acetaldehyde modified–hemoglobin was measured in patients admitted for drug and alcohol treatment. A positive correlation was found between the amount of reported drinking and percent acetaldehyde hemoglobin (0.055% in those who reported consuming more than six drinks per day vs 0.026% in those reporting fewer than six drinks per day). The cutoff of 0.03% had the best overall sensitivity (67%) and specificity of (77%).[27] Another study found that acetaldehyde–hemoglobin adducts showed promise as markers of alcohol abuse in women. The overall accuracy for detection of alcoholic women was higher than that of traditional markers of alcohol abuse: GGT, AST, ALT, and MCV.[28] Recently, a sensitive liquid chromatography (LC) coupled to time-of-flight mass spectrometry method was used to detect acetaldehyde-modified peptides after tryptic digestion of hemoglobin.[29] These researchers demonstrated that these acetaldehyde-modified hemoglobin peptides were elevated after recent alcohol consumption but declined rapidly during abstinence, reaching non–alcohol-user levels after 5 days. This suggests that this particular marker would be able to detect only relatively recent ethanol use.

Measurement of the levels of IgA antibodies directed against acetaldehyde-modified red cell proteins rather than the adducts themselves was found to have potential clinical value in distinguishing between abstainers and alcohol abusers (sensitivity 73% and specificity 94%).[26]

Quantification of acetaldehyde adducts or the IgAs directed against them are used primarily for research into the mechanism of alcohol-induced disease. A number of studies have reported sensitivity and specificity comparable to the better alcohol biomarkers in current clinical use. Nevertheless, further research into the utility of these biomarkers in a variety of clinical settings is needed to define their practicality for screening and diagnosis of alcohol use disorders.

Ethyl Glucuronide and Ethyl Sulfate

Ethyl glucuronide and ethyl sulfate are minor products of phase II ethanol metabolism (<0.1% of total ethanol disposition).[30,31] Ethyl glucuronide is formed through ethanol conjugation with activated glucuronic acid catalyzed by UDP-glucuronosyltransferase and ethyl sulfate through sulfotransferase-mediated conjugation of ethanol with sulfate.[30,32] There has been increasing interest in these markers because of their potential to detect recent ethanol use and their sensitivity to relatively low-level ethanol exposure.[33]

The presence of EtG and EtS in urine suggests recent alcohol consumption in a time frame when ethanol itself may no longer be measureable in breath or body fluids. EtG and EtS may be detected in urine for about 1 day after consumption of a dose of ethanol less than 0.25 g/kg and for 2 days after a dose of less than 50 g/kg.[32] EtG and EtS appear to be very sensitive markers of ethanol use. Consumption of a relatively small quantity of ethanol, 7 g (equivalent to the ethanol content of 0.33 L of 2.2% ethanol beer) may result in detectable EtG for as long as 6 hours in urine.[31] In another study, volunteers consumed low (0.25 g/kg), medium (0.50 g/kg), and high (0.75 g/kg) doses of ethanol. Using a cutoff for urine EtG of 100 ng/mL and a 24-hour testing point, only two thirds of the high- and medium-dose subjects and none of the low-dose subjects were positive.[35] The detection time in urine appears to be longer in heavy chronic ethanol users. EtG and EtS were measurable in the urine of alcohol-dependent patients for 2 to 5 days after admission for detoxification treatment. Both markers were found to have a similar detection window for heavy drinking.[32] The detection time in urine and sensitivity of EtG as an alcohol biomarker are therefore influenced by amount of ethanol consumed and the cutoff concentration of the analytical method. Because of these factors, it may not be possible to distinguish consumption of a single low-alcohol–content drink a few hours before collection from a major heavy drinking episode several days before collection, based solely on the concentration of EtG or EtS present.

There have been reports of false-positive urine EtG and EtS tests. It may possible for specimens to be positive due to sources of ethanol other than intentional consumption of alcohol-containing beverages, especially if low-level cutoffs are used. Common cutoffs offered by laboratories for EtG in urine are 100, 500, or 1000 ng/mL. The challenge is to choose a cutoff that would minimize false positives from incidental ethanol exposure, while still maintaining sensitivity to heavy recent intentional alcohol consumption. Several studies have demonstrated detectable EtG and EtS due to exposure to ethanol-containing consumer products such as mouthwash and hand sanitizer. After intensive use of a high-alcohol–content mouthwash, EtG and EtS were found in urine of some subjects, all at concentrations less than 500 ng/mL. It was concluded that setting a urine cutoff above 500 ng/mL would eliminate mouthwash as a source of false-positive results.[36] Frequent application of ethanol-containing hand sanitizer, as might occur with workers in a patient care facility, was found to cause elevations in EtG above 1000 ng/mL in some subjects. In this same study, EtS was detected in fewer subjects and at concentrations all less than 100 ng/mL.[37] The aforementioned reports suggest that even a cutoff of 1000 ng/mL for EtG, may not completely eliminate false-positive EtG urine tests due to unintentional alcohol exposure.

Another cause of potential clinical false positives is in vitro production of EtG in specimens containing ethanol and urinary tract pathogens. Formation of EtG (but not EtS) was demonstrated in urine specimens in the presence of ethanol and *Escherichia coli*.[38] In 2006, the United States Substance Abuse and Mental Health Services Administration (SAMHSA) issued an advisory because of concern related to false-positive EtG tests. This document contained a warning against the use of the EtG test as sole evidence in determining abstinence in criminal justice, regulatory, or legal settings.[1] EtG and/or EtS, however, may still have a valuable role in clinical setting where they can be used to monitor for compliance in alcohol abuse treatment programs and as a motivational tool to prevent relapse.[39,40] Patients in such programs, however, should be advised against use of food and health care products that contain ethanol.

On the other hand, false-negative EtG tests can occur as a result of bacterial hydrolysis, especially in specimens containing *Escherichia coli* (a common cause of urinary tract infection). The high levels of β-glucuronidase produced by this organism can hydrolyze the EtG present in the specimen, resulting in falsely low values. In contrast, EtS seems less subject to bacterial hydrolysis. Refrigeration or frozen storage is recommended to improve EtG stability in these specimens.[41]

A number of different analytical techniques have been used to measure EtG and EtS in urine. Immunoassay kits for EtG are now commercially available.[42] It is recommended that initially positive specimens by immunoassay be confirmed by more definitive methods if results are to be used for legal purposes. Such methods include HPLC/tandem mass spectrometry,[43] Liquid chromatography/mass spectrometry (LC/MS),[34,44] and capillary zone electrophoresis.[45]

PEth

PEth is an ethanol metabolite that has potential as a longer-term marker of ethanol consumption. It is a group of phospholipids formed through a phospholipase D–mediated reaction of ethanol with the phosphatidylcholine in cell membranes.[46–48] For clinical purposes, PEth is usually measured in whole blood. Most of the PEth in whole blood resides in red blood cell membranes and is eliminated from blood with a half-life of 4 days.[46,47]

A number of clinical studies have shown that PEth has a relatively long window of detection of prior ethanol use and is free of bias due to gender or liver disease. PEth was detectable in blood of alcohol detoxification patients for as long as 4 weeks after ethanol was last consumed (positive in 92.5% of patients after 1 week and 64.3% after 4 weeks of sobriety). Furthermore, PEth was measurable in more patients and for longer periods of time than other traditional markers, MCV, GGT, and % CDT.[49] The sensitivity (94.5%) and specificity (100%) of PEth was found to be comparable to FAEEs in hair and superior to that of % CDT, GGT, and MCV. There was also a significant correlation between PEth and the grams of ethanol consumed in the last 7 days.[50] No gender differences were observed.[49,51] A study of PEth in women of reproductive age showed it to be a sensitive indicator of moderate to heavy drinking in this population. Consequently this marker may have application in monitoring for alcohol use during pregnancy.[51] Furthermore, unlike many of the traditional alcohol markers, PEth concentration was not influenced by liver disease, suggesting that this marker may be useful in monitoring alcohol use in patients with liver disorders.[52] PEth may also be of value to screen patients for alcohol use disorders in clinical settings (ED), where patients may underreport the true extent of their alcohol use. In a study of nonintoxicated males presenting to the ED, about a third of those reporting no ethanol use during the last year and a third of those screening negative by a standardized questionnaire had positive PEth.[53] In a comparison of alcohol biomarkers for assessment of alcohol intake in alcohol-dependent patients, PEth was found to have a stronger correlation to amount of ethanol consumed and a superior diagnostic sensitivity (99%) than CDT (77%), GGT (44%), or MCV (40%). However, the combined CDT–GGT test had a similar sensitivity (94%) to that of PEth alone.[54]

In most of the earlier clinical studies, PEth was measured by HPLC with evaporative light-scattering detection.[47,49,50,53] This method measures PEth as a single entity even though PEth is actually a group of phospholipids. The structure of these lipids includes a phosphoethanol attached to two fatty acid moieties, which can vary in carbon chain lengths and number of double bonds. Consequently, many different PEth species are possible. There is increasing interest in studying the patterns of formation of these different PEth species in the blood of alcohol-dependent subjects. With the newer, sensitive LC/high-resolution MS[55] and LC/tandem-MS[56] methods, it is possible to identify and quantify these different PEth species. These methods, however, are expensive and require a high level of technical expertise. To increase the practical clinical use of PEth as an alcohol biomarker, an immunoassay method for PEth is under development.[48]

FAEEs

FAEEs are nonoxidative products of ethanol metabolism. They are formed in blood and other tissues through enzyme-mediated esterification of ethanol with fatty acids. These substances are gaining interest as biomarkers of ethanol use and have been evaluated in a number of different specimen types: blood,[57] hair,[58–66] and meconium.[59–73] FAEEs are measurable in blood soon after ethanol consumption and their levels decline rapidly within the first 24 hours. However, they can remain detectable in the blood of heavy drinkers for as long as 4 days after ethanol was last consumed.[57] Because of their relative short half-life and instability in blood, analyses of FAEEs are performed primarily on alternative specimen types such as hair and meconium. The FAEEs in hair are believed to originate from local production by the sebum glands.[58] The FAEE in meconium is of fetal, not maternal, origin. Ethanol consumed by the mother can cross the placenta but maternally produced FAEEs do not. Therefore, the FAEEs present in the fetus are derived from fetal production of these substances from ethanol.[59] Baseline studies, however, have shown trace amounts of FAEE in meconium of neonates from abstaining mothers. It is believed that this may occur as the result of FAEE formation from endogenous ethanol or from incidental ethanol exposure from common food additives and medications.[59] Therefore it is important to establish appropriate cutoffs for determination of clinically significant ethanol exposure taking these baseline values into consideration.

Hair and meconium specimens provide a long (several months) window of detection of ethanol use patterns. A number of studies have shown that levels of FAEEs in such specimens can be related to long-term heavy alcohol use. FAEE in hair was studied in subjects with different alcohol consumption habits (from abstainers to alcoholics) as well as in populations with different rates of alcohol use. Most studies reported that the amount of ethanol consumed could be related to FAEE levels in hair but it was not always possible to distinguish moderate social drinkers from abstainers. Consequently, this marker may be best applied to screen for and identify chronic heavy drinkers.[58-66]

FAEE testing of meconium is being utilized more commonly to screen neonates for intrauterine ethanol exposure. Investigators have evaluated meconium FAEE levels in specimens from different populations and various clinical settings.[59,67-70] Most studies were able to show a relationship between the levels of FAEE in meconium and the degree of alcohol exposure. Other investigators reported correlations of FAEE in meconium to clinical parameters. Higher rates of positive FAEE screens for alcohol exposure were found in infants born in high-risk obstetric units compared to infants born in the general population.[71] Increasing FAEE levels in meconium were related to poorer mental and psychomotor development in infants during their first 2 years of life.[72] These studies suggest that meconium screening may be an effective way to identify at risk infants, allowing for earlier intervention and treatment.

Measurement of FAEE in meconium and hair presents a number of challenging analytic considerations. The complex matrix of these specimens necessitates rigorous cleanup steps before analysis. Furthermore, there is a need to choose which FAEEs to quantitate from among the many different ones that have been identified in these specimens. For diagnostic purposes, the Society of Hair Testing Consensus document recommends that concentrations of four of these FAEEs (ethyl palmitate, ethyl myristate, ethyl oleate, and ethyl stearate) should be determined and reported as the combined sum.[74] However, there does not appear to be a consensus among investigators as to which FAEEs should be measured in meconium.[59] FAEEs in hair and meconium are most commonly measured by gas chromatography/mass spectrometry (GC/MS) after headspace solid-phase microextraction[60,61,63-66,68,71,73] or by LC-MS/MS.[67] An improved, sensitive automated procedure for FAEE meconium testing, suitable for prenatal alcohol screening, was recently described.[73]

ALTERNATIVE SPECIMEN TYPES

In addition to blood and urine, there has been active research into the feasibility of measuring alcohol biomarkers in other specimen types, such as hair, nails, meconium, and umbilical cord tissue. These specimens can be used to detect chronic prior ethanol consumption over a longer time frame (several months) than is feasible with serum or urine specimens (hours to a few weeks). Analyses of ethanol markers in hair or nail specimens for forensic death investigations provide a suitable alternative means to obtain premortem alcohol consumption information, especially when other specimen types are no longer retrievable or are degraded. Hair or nail alcohol biomarker determinations have additional clinical applications in monitoring of patients in substance abuse treatment programs, management of chronic diseases exacerbated by alcohol use, testing of employees in safety-sensitive positions, and as proof of long-term abstinence for legal purposes or restoration of driving privileges. Currently there is active investigation as to the feasibility of using these alternative specimen types for screening of mothers at risk for ethanol abuse during pregnancy and for identification of neonates that may have been exposed to ethanol prenatally.[4] Documentation of maternal ethanol use is one of the criteria for diagnosis of fetal alcohol spectrum disorders (FASD). Maternal hair or nail testing for alcohol markers has been utilized as part of intervention or prevention strategies for fetal alcohol syndrome (FAS) and fetal alcohol spectrum disorders (FASD).[63,75] Umbilical cord and meconium alcohol biomarker testing are potential tools for early recognition of alcohol-exposed infants, allowing for earlier treatment and potentially better clinical outcomes.

Hair and Nails

Measurement of EtG, EtS, and FAEEs in hair and nails has been proposed as a means of detecting heavy prior ethanol use. Recently, the Society of Hair Testing has published consensus guidelines regarding measurement of EtG and FAEE in hair.[74] This organization recommends that EtG be measured by LC/MS or LC/tandem MS (GC-MS/MS) and that FAEEs be analyzed by GC/MS after headspace solid-phase microextraction. The suggested cutoff for FAEE is 0.5 to 1.0 ng/mg, depending on length of proximal hair segment and for EtG, 30 pg/mg of scalp hair. Nevertheless, application of these cutoffs may result in some false positives or negatives, especially in individuals whose consumption of alcohol is at the borderline between social and excessive drinking. EtG or FAEE measurements are not biased by the natural hair color. However, the amount of these markers in hair may be falsely low or high due to use of certain hair care products or cosmetic treatments. Frequent washing or hair bleaching may reduce EtG and hair dyeing may decrease FAEE content of hair. Regular applications of high alcohol content hair care products may cause false positives for FAEEs.[63,75,76]

Hair analysis for EtG and FAEEs has been evaluated for a number of potential clinical applications. Studies have shown that heavy alcohol consumption could be indentified by analysis of both EtG and FAEE content of hair.[61-63,66] However, for alcoholics there was no clear correlation between EtG and FAEE levels in hair and self-reported EtOH consumption.[64,66] Owing to biological variability and individual differences in use of hair cosmetics, results may be difficult to interpret. Consequently, it is suggested that both markers be tested on the same hair specimens as a means to recognize false positives and negatives.[61,63,64] Hair FAEE screening has also been used to identify heavy maternal drinking in a population at risk for FASDs.[60] Testing of neonatal hair specimens for alcohol exposure is possible up to 3 months postpartum.[2]

Measurement of EtG in fingernail clippings has been studied as an alternative to hair analysis. Hair and nail EtG content was compared in paired specimens from the same individuals. It was found that the ETG content was significantly higher in nails than in the matching hair specimens. This suggests that it may be easier to detect and track EtG in nail specimens than in hair. Another potential advantage of nails over hair would be the fact that nails are not be subjected to the types of cosmetic treatments such as bleaching, which is known to lower hair EtG levels. It was concluded that nail clippings are a suitable specimen type for detection of EtG and may prove to be a superior to hair analysis.[75]

Meconium and Umbilical Cord

FAEEs and EtG have been measured in specimens from newborns as a means of detection of prenatal exposure to ethanol. Meconium and umbilical cord tissue have an advantage over other types of specimens in that they can be obtained noninvasively. Meconium is the first stool passed by the neonate, usually within the first 3 days of birth. Meconium starts forming in fetal gut from about week 20 of gestation. Consequently, this specimen should provide a means to detect intrauterine alcohol exposure during the latter half of pregnancy. Both temperature and light effect FAEE stability in meconium specimens.[69] Consequently, meconium should be kept frozen and protected from light before analysis. Similar to what was reported in maternal hair studies, combined measurement of FAEEs and EtG in meconium may provide a better evaluation of the degree of intrauterine ethanol exposure by reducing the number of false positives and negatives.[68]

Umbilical cord is another specimen that has been used to measure prenatal alcohol exposure. Umbilical cord tissue can be collected immediately after birth. This type of specimen is faster and easier to obtain than meconium. This tests is currently offered commercially at the U.S. Drug Testing Laboratories (USDTL). USDTL claims that cord tissue positive for PEth is an indication of heavy maternal ethanol consumption.[77] For EtG in umbilical cord tissue, the detection period is about 3 weeks before delivery. This is much shorter window of assessment for intrauterine ethanol than can be achieved with meconium testing.

SUMMARY

There is considerable ongoing interest in the development of sensitive and specific tests for the detection and management of alcohol use disorders. Several of the newer direct markers have potential in this regard. Further evaluation of these markers in different clinical settings and in different populations will help determine the clinical utility of these markers. Progress in this field requires development of improved analytical procedures. The lack of readily available automated methods to measure many of these markers impedes adoption of these tests for routine clinical use. As in any method development process, it is crucial to understand potential interfering substances and causes of false-positive and false-negative results. Further information is needed to establish appropriate cutoff concentrations for alcohol screening tests and to determine the relationship between a given marker concentration and the extent and duration of the patient's exposure to alcohol. Ultimately, studies need to be performed to determine whether or not the use of these markers improves clinical outcomes.

REFERENCES

1. Center for Substance Abuse Treatment. The role of biomarkers in the treatment of alcohol use disorders. Substance Abuse treatment Advisory 2006;5(4). Available at: http://www.kap.samhsa.gov/products/manuals/advisory/pdfs/0609_biomarkers.pdf. Accessed April 29, 2012.
2. Hannuksela M, Liisanatti M, Nissinen A, et al. Biochemical markers of alcoholism. Clin Chem Lab Med 2007;45(8):953–61.
3. Litten R, Bradley A, Moss H. Alcohol biomarkers in applied settings: recent advances and future research opportunities. Alcohol Clin Exp Res 2010;34(6):955–67.
4. Bakhireva LN, Savage DD. Focus on: biomarkers of fetal alcohol exposure and fetal alcohol effects. Alcohol Res Health 2011;34(1):56–63.

5. Substance Abuse and Mental Health Services Administration. Results from the 2010 National Survey on Drug Use and Health: summary of national findings, NSDUH Series H-41, HHS Publication No. (SMA) 11-4658. Rockville (MD): Substance Abuse and Mental Health Services Administration; 2011. Available at: http://www.samhsa.gov/data/NSDUH/2k10Results/Web/HTML/2k10Results.htm. Accessed April 29, 2012.

6. Centers for Disease Control and Prevention, National Center on Birth Defects and Developmental Disabilities, Division of Birth Defects and Developmental Disabilities. Data and statistics in the United States. In: Fetal alcohol spectrum disorders. Available at: http://www.cdc.gov/ncbddd/fasd/data.html. Accessed April 29, 2012.

7. Division of Population Health, National Center for Chronic Disease Prevention and Health Promotion Alcohol Use and Health. In: Alcohol and Public Health Fact Sheets. Available at: http://www.cdc.gov/alcohol/fact-sheets/alcohol-use.htm. Accessed April 29, 2012.

8. Schuckit MA. Ethanol and methanol. In: Brunton LL, Chabner BA, Knollmann BC, editors. Goodman & Gilman's The Pharmacological basis of therapeutics. 12th edition. New York: McGraw-Hill; 2011. Available at: http://www.accesmedicine.com/content.aplx?aID=16666094. Accessed March 30, 2012.

9. Tuma J, Casey C. Dangerous byproducts of alcohol breakdown: focus on adducts. Alcohol Res Health 2003;27(4):285–90.

10. Niemela O, Alatalo P. Biomarkers of alcohol consumption and related liver disease. Scand J Clin Lab Invest 2010;70:305–12.

11. Niemela O. Biomarkers in alcoholism. Clin Chim Acta 2007;377:39–49.

12. Das S, Dhanya L, Vasudevan D. Biomarkers of alcoholism: an updated review. Scand J Clin Lab Invest 2008;68:81–92.

13. Delanghe J, De Buyzere M. Carbohydrate deficient transferrin and forensic medicine. Clin Chim Acta 2009;406:1–7.

14. Allen J, Litten R, Fertig J, et al. Carbohydrate-deficient transferrin: an aid to early recognition of alcohol relapse. Am J Addict 2001;10(Suppl):24–8.

15. Helander A, Wielders J, Jeppsson J, et al. Toward standardization of carbohydrate-deficient transferrin (CDT) measurements: II. Performance of a laboratory network running the HPLC candidate reference measurement procedure and evaluation of a candidate reference material. Clin Chem Lab Med 2010;48(11):1585–92.

16. Sillanaukee P, Strid N, Allen J, et al. Possible reasons why heavy drinking increases carbohydrate-deficient transferrin. Alcohol Clin Exp Res 2001;25:34–40.

17. Golka K, Wiese A. Carbohydrate-deficient transferrin (CDT)—a biomarker for long-term alcohol consumption. J Toxicol Environ Health B 2004;7:319–37.

18. Flemming M, Anton R, Spies C. A review of genetic, biological, pharmacological, and clinical factors that affect carbohydrate-deficient transferrin levels. Alcohol Clin Exp Res 2004;28:1347–55.

19. Bergstrom J, Helander A. Influence of alcohol use, ethnicity, age, gender, BMI and smoking on the serum transferrin glycoform pattern: implications for use of carbohydrate-deficient transferrin (CDT) as alcohol biomarker. Clin Chim Acta 2008;388:59–67.

20. Koivisto H, Hietala J, Anttila P, et al. Long-term ethanol consumption and macrocytosis: diagnostic and pathogenic implications. J Lab Clin Med 2006;147(4):191–6.

21. Anton F. Carbohydrate-deficient transferrin for detection and monitoring of sustained heavy drinking. What have we learned? Where do we go from here? Alcohol 2001;25:184–8.

22. Hock B, Schwarz M, Domke I, et al. Validity of carbohydrate-deficient transferrin (%CDT), gamma-glutamyltransferase (GGT) and mean corpuscular volume (MCV) as biomarkers for chronic alcohol abuse: a study in patients with alcohol dependence and liver disorders of non-alcoholic and alcoholic origin. Addiction 2005; 100:1477–86.

23. Hietala J, Koivisto H, Anttila P, et al. Comparison of the combined marker GGT-CDT and the conventional laboratory markers of alcohol abuse in heavy drinkers, moderate drinkers and abstainers. Alcohol Alcohol 2006;41:528–33.

24. Setshedi M, Wands R, de la Monte S. Acetaldehyde adducts in alcoholic liver disease. Oxidat Med Cell Longev 2010;3(3):178–85.

25. Freeman T, Tuma D, Thiele G, et al. Recent advances in alcohol-induced adduct formation. Alcohol Clin Exp Res 2005;29(7):1310–6.

26. Hietala J, Kovisto H, Latvala J, et al. IgAs against acetetaldehyde-modified red cell protein as a marker of ethanol consumption in male alcoholic subjects, moderate drinkers, and abstainers. Alcohol Clin Exp Res 2006;30(10):1693–8.

27. Hazelett S, Liebelt R, Brown W, et al. Evaluation of acetaldehyde-modified hemoglobin and other markers of chronic heavy alcohol use: effects of gender and hemoglobin concentration. Alcohol Clin Exp Res 1998;22(4):1813–9.

28. Hurme L, Seppa K, Rajaniem H, et al. Chromatographically identified alcohol-induced haemoglobin adducts as markers of alcohol abuse among women. Eur J Clin Invest 1998;28:87–94.

29. Toennes A, Wagner M, Kauert G. Application of LC-TOF MS to analysis of hemoglobin acetaldehyde adducts in alcohol detoxification patients. Anal Bioanal Chem 2010; 398:769–77.

30. Dahl H, Stephanson N, Beck O, et al. Comparison of urinary excretion characteristics of ethanol and ethyl glucuronide. J Anal Toxicol 2002;26:201–4.

31. Wurst F, Dressen S, Allen J, et al. Ethyl sulphate: a direct ethanol metabolite reflecting recent alcohol consumption. Addiction 2006;101:204–11.

32. Helander A, Bottcher M, Fehr C, et al. Detection times for urinary ethyl glucuronide and ethyl sulfate in heavy drinkers during alcohol detoxification. Alcohol Alcohol 2009;44:55–61.

33. Jatlow P, O'Malley S. Clinical (nonforensic) application of ethyl glucuronide measurement: Are we ready? Alcohol Clin Exp Res 2010;34(6):968–75.

34. Stephenson N, Dahl H, Helander A, et al. Direct quantification of ethyl glucuronide in clinical urine samples by liquid chromatograph-mass spectrometry. Ther Drug Monit 2002;24(5):645–51.

35. Wojcik M, Hawthorne J. Sensitivity of commercial ethyl glucuronide (ETG) testing in screening for alcohol abstinence. Alcohol Alcohol 2007;42(4):317–20.

36. Reisfield G, Goldberger B, Pesce A, et al. Ethyl glucuronide, ethyl sulfate, and ethanol in urine after intensive exposure to high ethanol content mouthwash. J Anal Toxicol 2011;35:264–8.

37. Reisfield G, Goldberger B, Crews B, et al. Ethyl glucuronide, ethyl sulfate, and ethanol in urine after sustained exposure to ethanol-based hand sanitizer. J Anal Toxicol 2011;335:85–91.

38. Helander A, Olsson I, Dahl H. Postcollection synthesis of ethyl glucuronide by bacteria in urine may cause false identification of alcohol consumption. Clin Chem 2007; 53(10):1855–7.

39. Skipper G, Weinmann W, Thierauf A, et al. Ethyl glulcuronide: a biomarker to identify alcohol use by health professionals recovering from substance use disorders. Alcohol Alcohol 2004;39(5):445–9.

40. Dahl H, Carlsson A, Hillgren K. et al. Urinary ethyl glucuronide and ethyl sulfate testing for detection of recent drinking in an outpatient treatment program for alcohol and drug dependence. Alcohol Alcohol 2011;46(3):278–82.

41. Helander A, Dahl H. Urinary tract infection: a risk factor for false-negative urinary ethyl glucuronide but not ethyl sulfate in the detection of recent alcohol consumption. Clin Chem 2005;51:1728–30.

42. Bottcher M, Beck O, Helander A. Evaluation of a new immunoassay for urinary ethyl glucuronide testing. Alcohol Alcohol 2008;43(1):46–8.
43. Beyer J, Vo T, Gerostamoulos D, et al. Validated method for the determination of ethylglucuronide and ethylsulfate in human urine. Anal Bioanal Chem 2011;400: 189–96.
44. Favretto D, Nalesso A, Frison G, et al. A novel and effective analytical approach for the LC-MS determination of ethyl glucuronide and ethyl sulfate in urine. Int J Legal Med 2010;124:161–4.
45. Jung B, Caslavska J, Thormann W. Determination of ethyl sulfate in human serum and urine by capillary zone electrophoresis. J Chromatogr A 2008;1206:26–32.
46. Hansson P, Caron M, Johnson G, et al. Blood phosphatidylethanol as a marker of alcohol abuse: levels in alcoholic males during withdrawal. Alcohol Clin Exp Res 1997;21(1):108–10.
47. Varga A, Hansson P, Johnson G, et al. Normalization rate and cellular localization of phosphatidylethanol in whole blood from chronic alcoholics. Clin Chim Acta 2000; 299:141–50.
48. Nissinen A, Makela S, Vuoristo J, et al. Immunological detection of in vitro formed phosphatidylethanol—an alcohol biomarker-with monoclonal antibodies. Alcohol Clin Exp Res 2008;32(6):921–7.
49. Wurst M, Thon N, Aradottir S, et al. Phosphatidylethanol: normalization during detoxification, gender aspects and correlation with other biomarkers and self-reports. Addict Biol 2010;15:88–95.
50. Hartmann S, Aradottir S, Graf M, et al. Phosphatidylethanol as a sensitive and specific biomarker-comparison with gamma-glutamyl transpeptidase, mean corpuscular volume and carbohydrate-deficient transferrin. Addict Biol 2006;12:81–4.
51. Stewart S, Law T, Randall P, et al. Phosphatidylethanol and alcohol consumption in reproductive age women. Alcohol Clin Exp Res 2010;34(3):488–92.
52. Stewart S, Reuben A, Brzezinski W, et al. Preliminary evaluation of phosphatidylethanol and alcohol consumption in patients with liver disease and hypertension. Alcohol Alcohol 2009;44(5):464–7.
53. Kip M, Spies C, Neumann T, et al. The usefulness of direct ethanol metabolites in assessing alcohol intake in nonintoxicated male patients in an emergency room setting. Alcohol Clin Exp Res 2008;32(7):1284–91.
54. Aradottir S, Gulber A, Gjerss S, et al. Phosphatidylethanol (PEth) concentrations in blood are correlated to reported alcohol intake in alcohol-dependent patients. Alcohol Alcohol 2006;41(4):431–7.
55. Nalesso A, Viel G, Cecchetto G, et al. Quantitative profiling of phosphatidylethanol molecular species in human blood by liquid chromatography high resolution mass spectrometry. J. Chromatogr. A 2011;1218:8423–31.
56. Zheng Y, Beck O, Helander A. Method development for routine liquid chromatography-mass spectrometry measurement of the alcohol biomarker phosphatidylethanol (PEth) in blood. Clin Chim Acta 2011;412:1428–35.
57. Borucki K, Dierkes J, Wartberg J, et al. In heavy drinkers, fatty acid ethyl esters remain elevated for up to 99 hours. Alcohol Clin Exp Res 2007;31(3):423–7.
58. Auwarter V, Sporkert F, Hartwig S, et al. Fatty acid ethyl esters in hair as markers of alcohol consumption: segmental hair analysis of alcoholics, social drinkers, and teetotalers. Clin Chem 2001;47(12):2114–23.
59. Chan D, Caprara D, Blanchette P, et al. Recent developments in meconium and hair testing methods for the confirmation of gestational exposures to alcohol and tobacco smoke. Clin Biochem 2004;37:429–38.

60. Kulaga V, Pragst F, Fulga N, et al. Hair analysis of fatty acid ethyl esters in the detection of excessive drinking in the context of fetal alcohol spectrum disorders. Ther Drug Monit 2009;31(2):262–5.
61. Hastedt M, Herre S, Pragst F, et al. Workplace alcohol testing program by combined use of ethyl glucuronide and fatty acid ethyl esters in hair. Alcohol Alcohol 2012;47(2): 127–32.
62. Pragst F, Rothe M, Moench B, et al. Combined use of fatty acid ethyl esters and ethyl glucuronide in hair for diagnosis of alcohol abuse: interpretation and advantages. Forensic Sci Int 2010;196:101–10.
63. Pragst F, Yegles M. Determination of fatty acid ethyl esters (FAEE) and ethyl glucuronide (EtG) in hair: a promising way for retrospective detection of alcohol abuse during pregnancy? Ther Drug Monit 2008;30:255–63.
64. Susse S, Selavka C, Mieczkowski T, et al. Fatty acid ethyl ester concentrations in hair and self-reported alcohol consumption in 644 cases from different origin. Forensic Sci Int 2010;196:111–7.
65. Wurst F, Alexson S, Wolfersdorf M, et al. Concentration of fatty acid ethyl esters in hair of alcoholics: comparison to other biological state markers and self reported-ethanol intake. Alcohol Alcohol 2004;39(1):33–8.
66. Yegles M, Labarthe A, Auwarter V, et al. Comparison of ethyl glucuronide and fatty acid ethyl ester concentrations in hair of alcoholics, social drinkers and teetotalers. Forensic Sci Int 2004;145:167–73.
67. Pichini S, Pellegrini M, Gareri J, et al. Liquid chromatography-tandem mass spectrometry for fatty acid ethyl esters in meconium: assessment of prenatal exposure to alcohol in two European cohorts. J Pharmaceut Biomed Anal 2008;48:927–33.
68. Bakdash A, Burger P, Goecke T, et al. Quantification of fatty acid ethyl esters (FAEE) and ethyl glucuronide (EtG) in meconium from newborns for detection of alcohol abuse in a maternal health evaluation study. Anal Bioanal Chem 2010;396:2469–77.
69. Moore C, Jones J, Lewis D. Prevalence of fatty acid ethyl esters in meconium specimens. Clin Chem 2003;49(1):133–6.
70. Bearer C, Santiago L, O'Riordan M, et al. Fatty acid ethyl esters: quantitative biomarkers for maternal alcohol consumption. J Pediatr 2005;146:824–30.
71. Goh Y, Hutson J, Lum L, et al. Rates of fetal alcohol exposure among newborns in a high-risk obstetric unit. Alcohol 2010;44:629–34.
72. Peterson J, Kirchner H, Xue W, et al. Fatty acid ethyl esters in meconium are associated with poorer neurodevelopmental outcomes to two years of age. J Pediatr 2008;152:788–92.
73. Hutson J, Rao C, Fulga N, et al. An improved method for rapidly quantifying fatty acid ethyl esters in meconium suitable for prenatal alcohol screening. Alcohol 2010;45: 193–9.
74. Society of Hair Testing. Consensus of the Society of Hair Testing on hair testing for chronic excessive alcohol consumption. Available at: http://www.soht.org/pdf/Revised%20Alcohol%20marker%20Consensus.pdf. Accessed April 30, 2012.
75. Jones J. Jones M, Plate C, et al. Liquid chromatography-tandem mass spectrometry assay to detect ethyl glucuronide in human fingernail: comparison to hair and gender differences. Am J Anal Chem 2012;3:83–91.
76. Hartwig S, Auwarter V, Pragst F. Effect of hair care and hair cosmetics as markers of chronically elevated alcohol consumption. Forensic Sci Int 2003;131:90–7.
77. U.S. Drug Testing Laboratories (USDTL). EtOH, a new alcohol biomarker that tests at risk newborns for heavy exposure to alcohol in utero. In: Testing services. Available at: http//www.usdtl.com/cordstatsetohm.html. Accessed April 14, 2012.

Drug Abuse
Newly-Emerging Drugs and Trends

Gregory G. Davis, MD, MSPH[a,b,]*

KEYWORDS

- Bath salts • Synthetic cannabinoids • Piperazine • Salvia • Kratom

KEY POINTS

- Various new drugs of abuse that are not yet regulated are available for purchase at stores and over the internet.
- Drugs with new chemical structures may be missed on routine drug screens that are not designed to detect them.
- Bath salts labeled "not for human consumption" are amphetamine analogs that cause cardiac, neurologic, and psychiatric symptoms characteristic for amphetamines.
- Herbal incense blends labeled "not for human consumption" contain synthetic cannabinoids that are more potent than marijuana.
- The incidence of drug abuse in the elderly is increasing and is projected to double by 2020.

The business of producing and selling illicit drugs of abuse is subject to the laws of commerce just as surely as any legitimate business. Specific drugs go in and out of fashion based on consumer demand, price, and availability. The promise of something new and improved appeals to drug users just as it does to people shopping for a new car. Legal efforts to control or eradicate drugs of abuse affect the price, availability, and profitability of a given drug. One approach drug traffickers can take to law enforcement efforts is to overwhelm police and customs officials with the volume of drug being sold; this is the approach of traffickers in cocaine or heroin. Another approach, which requires a degree of sophistication in chemistry, is to create

Disclosure: The author has no relationship with a commercial company that has a direct financial interest in the subject of this article, in the materials discussed within this article, or with a competitor to any company or substance discussed in this article.

[a] Forensic Division, Department of Pathology, University of Alabama at Birmingham, 1515 Sixth Avenue South, Room 220, Birmingham, AL 35233-1601, USA; [b] Jefferson County Coroner/Medical Examiner Office, 1515 Sixth Avenue South, Room 220 Birmingham, Alabama 35233-1601, USA

* Forensic Division, Department of Pathology, University of Alabama at Birmingham, 1515 Sixth Avenue South, Room 220, Birmingham, AL 35233-1601.

E-mail address: gdavis@uab.edu

Table 1
Emerging drugs of abuse

Name	Alternate Names	Effect	Chemical Analog	Clinical Effects
Bath salts	Charge Plus Cloud 9 Hurricane Charlie Ivory Wave Ocean Snow Red Dove Scarface White Dove White Lightning White Rush (many more exist)	Stimulant	Amphetamine	Hypertension Tachycardia Dysrhythmia Myocardial Infarct Seizures Tremors Psychosis Paranoia
Legal ecstasy	Benzo fury Exotic super strong Head rush MDAI party pills XXX Strong as Hell (others exist)	Stimulant	Piperazine	Tachycardia Palpitations Prolonged QT Interval Headache Seizures Anxiety
Mephentermine	Potenay Potemax	Stimulant	Amphetamine	Same as for bath salts
Herbal incense	Black Magic Cloud 9 K2 Smoke Spice Diamond Spice Gold (many more exist)	Hallucinogen	Cannabinoids	Supraventricular Tachycardia Seizures Psychosis Paranoia
Methoxetamine	None found	Hallucinogen	Ketamine	Tachycardia Hypertension Nystagmus Confusion Dissociation

Salvia	Diviners Sage
	Magic Mint
	Maria pastora
	Purple Sticky
	Sally D
		Hallucinogen	Salvinorin A	Hallucinations (seldom
				  present for medical
				  evaluation)

Kratom	Ithang Kakuam Ketum Krypton Thom	Opiate	Mitragynine	Low dose – stimulant High dose – opiate effect
Xylazine	Anestesia de Caballo	Tranquilizer	Xylazine	Skin ulcers

Note. Street names for herbal incense and kratom obtained from reports and user experience pages at http://www.erowid.com.

new, more potent compounds that evade existing laws by virtue of their novel chemical structures. These new drugs are chemical variations of existing stimulants, hallucinogens, or opiates. This article gives an overview of these new drugs of abuse, which are listed in **Table 1**. (Subsequent articles in this issue discuss bath salts and synthetic cannabinoids in greater detail.) This article also presents some new trends in drug abuse, as well as some resources for investigating or learning about trends that will develop in the future.

STIMULANTS
Bath Salts

Amphetamine is a traditional backbone for chemical alteration of side groups, leaving the stimulant or mood-altering effects intact while avoiding laws against existing drugs. The products of this chemical tinkering became known as "designer drugs" in the 1980's.[1] The current manifestation of this practice is being sold as "bath salts," one of many street names for various amphetamine analogs.[2] These bath salts are sold at stores[2] or over the internet[3] and were first found in the United States in 2009.[4] Purchasers know perfectly well that they are buying stimulant drugs promoted in a way designed to skirt laws and avoid legislative interference.[3] Bath salts bear a prominent label stating "not for human consumption" to hide the true nature of the product and as a means of avoiding regulation by the US Food and Drug Administration.[4] Bath salts are attractive to users because the product is cheap (about $20),[2] powerful, and likely to escape detection on a standard drug screen.[4]

Bath salts are hardly a pure product, and they can contain 1 or more active ingredients. Two common ingredients are 3,4-methylenedioxypyrovalerone and 4-methylcathinone (mephedrone, similar to the cathinone that naturally occurs in the leaves of khat).[4] Whatever the exact chemical nature of the compounds in bath salts, they act as amphetamine analogs, altering the proper transmission of dopamine, norepinephrine, and serotonin.[4] As amphetamine analogs, the components of bath salts can produce undesirable cardiac, neurologic, and psychiatric side effects up to and including death. [3]

The number of bath salt–related calls to US poison control centers increased from 303 in 2010 to 4720 by August 31, 2011. Most of these calls were related to tachycardia, hypertension, agitation, hallucinations, extreme paranoia, and delusions. Anecdotal reports from patients seen for emergency medical evaluation are in keeping with adverse side effects of amphetamines, namely, myocardial infarction or dysrhythmias, seizures or tremors, and psychosis or paranoia.[4] Bath salt use should be considered in the differential diagnosis of any individual not known to have a psychiatric disorder who presents with bizarre behavior. Benzodiazepines are an appropriate treatment to calm agitated persons and stop seizures in patients presenting with bath salt intoxication[4] as are cardiac rhythm monitoring and any necessary supportive measures.[5]

Piperazine Derivatives

Piperazine and related compounds have effects similar to amphetamines and have been used as stimulants in clubs or at rave parties. The premier example of this drug family is 1-benzylpiperazine (BZP or A2), and this compound has been controlled in the United States as a schedule I substance since 2004. Other piperazine analogs, however, are not controlled substances. BZP inhibits serotonin reuptake and inhibits serotonin transport.[5]

Piperazine derivatives are usually sold as a mixture of several different compounds. The onset of action takes about 2 hours, so inexperienced users may take more pills thinking that the drug has not worked. These drugs cause palpitations, headache, tachycardia, and anxiety. Seizures and QT prolongation have been reported, the latter in 32% of patients studied. [5]

Treatment is supportive, and cardiac rhythm monitoring is appropriate. Commercially available drug screens have variable success at detecting various piperazine derivatives.[5]

HALLUCINOGENS

Articles report abuse of new chemical variants of cannabinoids or ketamine. Of these, the synthetic cannabinoids are more common in the United States.

Synthetic Cannabinoids

Synthetic cannabinoids first appeared in the United States in 2008.[4] Examples of synthetic cannabinoids are K2 or Spice; these products are sold as herbal blend incense not intended for human consumption, but people are buying this "incense" as a legal alternative to marijuana.[6] The cannabinoids added to these herbal blends have been synthesized chemically rather than being derived from cannabinoids that occur naturally in the hemp plant (*Cannabis sativa*).[4] Because the synthetic cannabinoids are chemically distinct from delta-9-tetrahydrocannabinol (THC), the main active ingredient in marijuana, it is more likely that these novel compounds will escape detection on drug screens, a feature attractive to users.[6]

THC acts as a partial agonist on endogenous CB1 cannabinoid receptors, producing altered consciousness, euphoria, relaxation, cognitive impairment, and increased reaction times. Partial agonists exhibit a plateau effect, beyond which no additional amount of drug increases the effect. Synthetic cannabinoids are full agonists, however, so a greater dose leads to a greater effect without any plateau. The duration of action of the synthetic cannabinoids may be longer than for THC or shorter, but the effect is more intense. Synthetic cannabinoids have been associated with seizures, supraventricular tachycardia, psychosis, and paranoid delusions.[4] The US Drug Enforcement Agency has now banned some of the synthetic cannabinoids in these products, but enterprising chemists have introduced new synthetic cannabinoids, and production and sale of these products continue.[6] Treatment for symptoms related to synthetic cannabinoid use is supportive; benzodiazepines are appropriate means of controlling agitation and anxiety.[5]

Methoxetamine

Methoxetamine is a congener of ketamine and phencyclidine (PCP), easily purchased via the internet.[7] Methoxetamine has a longer duration of action and greater intensity of effects than ketamine.[8] Few countries regulate methoxetamine[9]; no restriction on methoxetamine currently exists in the United States.[7] Case reports from the United States[7] and from Switzerland[9] describe individual cases of intoxication with methoxetamine. In each case, the methoxetamine intoxication caused tachycardia, hypertension, confusion, dissociation, and nystagmus, findings similar to the pharmacologic effects of ketamine. Supportive care led to full recovery in each case.

OPIATE ANALOGS

Opium derivatives and analogs are a perennial drug of abuse. Several different preparations can be used as alternatives to commonly available opiates.

Salvia

Salvia divinorum is a species of mint that contains a psychoactive compound, salvinorin A. Salvia is becoming increasingly popular as a hallucinogen in the United States, but it is classified here with the opiate analogs because salvinorin A is a kappa opioid receptor agonist with a short duration. Kappa opioid receptor stimulation leads to hallucinations and spinal anesthesia but does not cause respiratory depression.[5] The leaves of salvia can be chewed or smoked. An extraction of salvinorin A is available via the internet as either an enhanced dried leaf product or as a tincture for oral use. Head shops sell salvia under various names as shown in **Table 1**.[10] Users rarely present for medical evaluation, given the short duration of action of the drug. Medical management consists of providing supportive care and benzodiazepines if needed to control agitation.[5]

Kratom

Kratom is a plant native to Southeast Asia, where it has long been used as an herbal drug. Kratom contains the alkaloid mitragynine, which is a mu-receptor opioid agonist. Kratom and a related preparation called *krypton* are available through the internet. Kronstrand and colleagues[11] reported 9 deaths in Sweden after use of Kratom purchased over the internet. They found that O-desmethyltramadol, an active metabolite of tramadol, had been added to the kratom to augment its opiate effects, and they warn that kratom is not as harmless as the Websites that promote it claim.

Mitragynine acts as a stimulant at low doses and as an opiate central nervous system depressant at high doses. Given the opiate effects and the possibility of the addition of other opiates to the substance medical management requires consideration of establishing a protected airway if respiratory depression is a concern. Naloxone can counteract the opiate effects but will not necessarily control seizures if they develop.[5]

New Opioid Medications

Pharmacologic opiate medications remain a more common drug of abuse than salvia or kratom. Price, availability, and the likelihood of legal repercussions, such as confrontations with police, affect the drug of choice in a given region.[12] In the author's jurisdiction, the common opiate of choice has ranged from propoxyphene to oxycodone to methadone to heroin over the last decade. An opiate currently unfamiliar in a given region may become the next opiate of choice tomorrow. Buprenorphine, for example, is an unusual opiate of abuse in the United States but the most common opiate of abuse in Finland.[12] Yokell and coworkers[12] also make the important point that opiate abusers often use their opiate in combination with a benzodiazepine, which reportedly enhances the sense of euphoria; but this combination is also more likely to lead to an overdose.[12]

New opiate formulations have the disadvantage of high cost, but they may be easier, and seem safer, for personnel in the medical, dental, or veterinary professions to obtain. Abnormal behavior or an unexpected death in one of these health care professionals may be caused by opiate abuse, and routine drug screens may not detect infrequently encountered opiates for which the screens are not designed.

VETERINARY DRUGS

Veterinary practices have access to drugs that are not approved for human use. In some cases, humans have begun abusing veterinary medications. Torruella[13] reports that xylazine has become a drug of abuse in Puerto Rico. Xylazine is a nonopiate tranquilizing agent that has been used in Puerto Rico as an adulterant in other drugs. A xylazine user interviewed by Torruella[13] reports that xylazine was originally used to cut heroin, but that in time some heroin addicts in Puerto Rico came to prefer the mixture of heroin and xylazine to pure heroin. Puerto Rican users have brought their xylazine habit with them to the mainland (Philadelphia, New York City). The distribution of xylazine abuse and the effects of chronic abuse are unknown, but users are particular prone to painful, oozing skin ulcers that do not necessarily arise only at sites of injection.[13]

De Oliveira and coworkers[14] report abuse of mephentermine, a veterinary drug in Brazil that has been diverted into the illicit drug market for abuse. Mephentermine is related to amphetamine, and so it has the potential to cause hypertension, cardiovascular disease, and sudden cardiac death.[14]

NEW MARKETS

A United States market once largely closed to drug use is beginning to open up—the elderly. Wu and Blazer[15] found a much higher rate of illicit drug use and prescription medication abuse in the Baby Boom generation, persons 50 to 64 years of age, compared with adults 65 years of age and older. The abuse of illicit and prescription drugs is increasing in the elderly, whereas ethanol-only abuse is decreasing. The drugs abused by this older cohort are primarily marijuana, opiates, or cocaine. Drug abuse among those 50 years of age or older is expected to double by 2020, in part because the number of people that age will increase and in part because that cohort is more likely to use drugs than the generation that preceded it. Most of the older drug users (70% to 90%) began using drugs earlier in life, but some begin drug use at this older age. Older adults are less likely than younger adults to perceive substance abuse as a problem and are unlikely to seek treatment.[15]

In light of the increasing incidence of drug abuse in the elderly, it is worth noting that old age brings with it changes in the metabolism and effects of drugs on the body. Drug metabolism decreases with increasing age. The most consistent finding is a decrease in the rate of P-450 metabolism, which slows the breakdown of chlordiazepoxide (Librium) and meperidine (Demerol). Glucuronidation seems unaffected by age. Blood flow to the liver decreases with age by roughly 30% to 50%, so elders have a decreased rate of clearance of drugs metabolized in the liver. Morphine, for example, is extensively metabolized on its first pass through the liver. Therefore, a decrease in blood flow to the liver of 30% to 50% decreases the rate of clearance of morphine by 30% to 50%.[16]

In addition to a decrease in the rate of drug metabolism with age, elders are more sensitive than younger adults to the effects of benzodiazepines, not only to the sedative effects but also to the side effect of respiratory depression. In a similar manner, the elderly are more sensitive to opiate and anesthetic agents than they were in their youth.[16] This increased sensitivity to benzodiazepines and opiates makes the elderly particularly susceptible to an overdose, especially if the 2 different medications are used concurrently. Elders taking benzodiazepines or opiates are also at increased risk of falling, whether they take the medications as prescribed or abuse them.[16]

INTERNET RESOURCES

The internet has drastically changed the world of drug trafficking and drug abuse. It should be obvious from this article alone that drug sellers and users constantly work to stay a step ahead of the law. It is difficult to report on a new drug phenomenon in the scientific literature quickly enough for the report to be relevant. What the internet lacks in peer review it makes up for in speed. Instant access to new drug information is available by entering a term into a search engine and reading representative Web pages found by the search. Three websites are described below that offer information particularly helpful in keeping up with newly emerging drugs of abuse.

www.bluelight.ru

This site is a discussion forum for drug users. The users describe their experience with a drug, how they used the drug (sometimes in explicit detail such as body mass of the user and the milligrams of drug used) and whether the drug provided the effect they had been seeking. Bluelight now has a presence on Facebook and a Twitter feed. Other similar sites exist.

www.erowid.com

This site bills itself as an online library of information about psychoactive plants, chemicals, and related topics. The site's stated aim is to provide information without judgment. The site accepts submissions from users, parents of users, health professionals, therapists, chemists, researchers, teachers, and attorneys. Erowid acts as a publisher of new information as well as a library for documents published elsewhere, such as selected abstracts from PubMed.

http://ww2.drugabuse.gov/about/organization/CEWG/CEWGHome.html

This site is maintained by the National Institute on Drug Abuse. The Community Epidemiology Work Group represents 20 cities and states across the United States. Members meet twice a year to compare their experience with drug abuse in their own region, with the intent of detecting new trends in drug abuse. The Community Epidemiology Work Group prepares publications of its findings; these publications are freely available over the Web site.

INCOMPREHENSIBLE OCCURRENCES

However diligently one attempts to learn about substances being abused, drug users can create scenarios one could never anticipate. As an example, the author's office investigated the death of an intravenous drug abuser who found a vial of insulin at the residence of a friend who had insulin-dependent diabetes mellitus. The abuser asked what was in the vial. When he was told that the substance was insulin, he said that he was willing to shoot up anything, whereupon he drew up a quantity of insulin and injected it intravenously. Shortly thereafter he was dead. No diligent study or Web site review would help one predict the circumstances of a case such as this; it is nonsensical. In such a setting, a physician is somewhat dependent on instinct, but mostly the physician is dependent on accurate history, something drug users and their friends are often loathe to provide.

SUMMARY

Existing screening tests are designed to detect known drugs; a previously unknown drug may escape detection. This, coupled with evasion of laws against misuse of established compounds, is the point of altering side groups to form a new drug with a potency similar to, or greater than, existing substances controlled by law.[17] The drug business is risky and potentially lucrative. Successful traffickers and users of drugs are wary, audacious, and resourceful, and the internet has become their essential field of play. Information remains freely available to all on the internet, helping addicts find new drugs and new sources of drugs. The internet can also provide information quickly to physicians treating belligerent addicts under the influence of some new substance. Finally, practicing physicians can expect to encounter drug abuse more commonly in the elderly as the Baby Boomer generation enters old age. Drug effects are often magnified in the elderly because of decreased metabolism and increased sensitivity to drugs with increasing age.

ACKNOWLEDGMENTS

The author thanks Edward W. Boyer, PhD, MD, Medical Toxicologist at the University of Massachusetts Medical School Department of Emergency Medicine, for suggestions and insights.

REFERENCES

1. Buchanan JF, Brown CR. 'Designer drugs'. A problem in clinical toxicology. Med Toxicol Adverse Drug Exp 1988;3:1–17.
2. Emergency department visits after use of a drug sold as "bath salts" – Michigan, November 13, 2010-March 31, 2011. MMWR Morb Mortal Wkly Rep 2011;60: 624–7.
3. Prosser JM, Nelson LS. The toxicology of bath salts: a review of synthetic cathinones. J Med Toxicol 2012;8:33–42.
4. Jerry J, Collins G, Streem D. Synthetic legal intoxicating drugs: The emerging 'incense' and 'bath salt' phenomenon. Cleve Clin J Med 2012;79:258–64.
5. Rosenbaum CD, Carreiro SP, Babu KM. Here today, gone tomorrow . . . and back again? A review of herbal marijuana alternatives (K2, Spice), synthetic cathinones (bath salts), Kratom, Salvia divinorum, methoxetamine, and piperazines. J Med Toxicol 2012;8:15–32.
6. Hu X, Primack BA, Barnett TE, et al. College students and the use of K2: an emerging drug of abuse in young persons. Subst Abuse Treat Prev Policy 2011;6:16.
7. Ward J, Rhyee S, Plansky J, et al. Methoxetamine: a novel ketamine analog and growing health-care concern. Clin Toxicol (Phila) 2011;49:874–5.
8. Corazza O, Schifano F, Simonato P, et al. Phenomenon of new drugs on the internet: the case of ketamine derivative methoxetamine. Hum Psychopharmacol 2012;27: 145–9.
9. Hofer KE, Grager B, Müller DM, et al. Ketamine-like effects after recreational use of methoxetamine. Ann Emerg Med 2012;60(1):97–9.
10. Lange JE, Reed MB, Croff JMK, et al. College student use of Salvia divinorum. Drug Alcohol Depend 2008;94:263–6.
11. Kronstrand R, Roman M, Thelander G, et al. Unintentional fatal intoxications with mitragynine and O-desmethyltramadol from the herbal blend Krypton. J Anal Toxicol 2011;35:242–7.
12. Yokell MA, Zaller ND, Green TC, et al. Buprenorphine and buprenorphine/naloxone diversion, misuse, and illicit use: an international review. Curr Drug Abuse Rev 2011;4:28–41.
13. Torruella RA. Xylazine (veterinary sedative) use in Puerto Rico. Subst Abuse Treat Prev Policy 2011;6:7.
14. De Oliveira MF, de Sousa HF, Lima MCD, et al. Mephentermine: rediscovering its biology and use, misuse and their implications. Rev Bras Psiquiatr 2011;33:98–9.
15. Wu L-T, Blazer DG. Illicit and nonmedical drug use among older adults: a review. J Aging Health 2011;23:481–504.
16. Hilmer Sarah N, Ford Gary A. General principles of pharmacology. In: Halter JB, Ouslander JG, Tinetti ME, et al, editors. Hazzard's geriatric medicine and gerontology. 6th edition. Available at: http://www.accessmedicine.com/content.aspx?aID=5107787. Accessed May 21, 2011.
17. Peters FT, Martinez-Ramirez JA. Analytical toxicology of emerging drugs of abuse. Ther Drug Monit 2010;32:532–9.

Bath Salts

Roy R. Gerona, PhD,[a,b],* and Alan H.B. Wu, PhD[a,c]

KEYWORDS

- Bath salts • Synthetic cathinones • Designer drugs • Mephedrone • MDPV

KEY POINTS

- Use of "bath salts" is attractive to young adults largely because of their stimulatory and hallucinogenic properties.
- Synthetic cathinones are the major components of bath salts but other classes of designer amines have also been incorporated in second-generation "legal high" or bath salts products.
- There are four major reactions involved in the metabolism of synthetic cathinones but the major metabolic pathway utilized vary among the different classes of synthetic cathinones.
- Rapid changes in the composition of bath salts pose tremendous challenge in the development of targeted methods for its laboratory analysis; high resolution mass spectrometry is well-suited to respond to this challenge.

INTRODUCTION

Since 2008, there have been increasing reports on fatal intoxications associated with the use of a new class of designer drugs called "bath salts." These products usually come in packets containing bags, tubes, or capsules of white to light brown powder carrying the warning "not for human consumption." They have also been marketed as "legal highs," plant foods, or insect repellents and can be easily purchased from Internet Web sites, smoke shops, and convenience stores. Analysis of their drug contents revealed that synthetic cathinones are their major components, although other classes of designer drugs such as aminoindanes, benzofurans, and piperazines may sometimes be incorporated. Generally, bath salts are regarded as stimulants and drug users exploit them as substitutes for methamphetamine and methylenedioxymethylamphetamine (MDMA). As

The authors have nothing to disclose.
[a] Department of Laboratory Medicine, University of California, San Francisco, San Francisco General Hospital, 1001 Potrero Avenue, San Francisco, CA 94110, USA; [b] San Francisco General Hospital, San Francisco, CA, USA; [c] Clinical Chemistry Division, San Francisco General Hospital, San Francisco, CA, USA
* Corresponding author. Department of Laboratory Medicine, University of California, San Francisco, 1001 Potrero Ave., San Francisco, CA 94110.
E-mail address: Roy.Gerona@ucsf.edu

such, intoxications seen in patients from bath salts use mimic or exaggerate symptoms seen in intoxications associated with amphetamines and its derivatives.[1–3]

REGULATORY LEGISLATION

In the United States, enforcement of federal drug laws is under the auspices of the Drug Enforcement Agency (DEA), a branch of the U.S. Department of Justice. Under the Control Substances of 1970, the DEA, together with the U.S. Food and Drug Administration (FDA), maintains a list of "Controlled Substances," consisting of five classifications or "schedules." In Schedule I, the drug or substance has a high potential for abuse, has no currently acceptable medical use for treatment of patients, and there is a lack of acceptable safety. As such, there can be no prescriptions written for use of these substances for medical purposes. Substances in DEA Schedules II to V list have medical uses and can be ordered by physicians via a prescription. Researchers can obtain a license for controlled substances for the purposes of analytical analysis.

In February of 2012, Senator Charles Schumer of New York proposed a national ban on the chemicals used in bath salts. At the time of his proposal, some 33 states had already put into place some measures to control the use and possession of these substances. The DEA announced in September 7, 2011 of their intention of using their emergency authority to ban chemicals contained in bath salts citing "imminent hazard" to the general public. On October 21, 2011, enacted the ban of mephedrone, 3,4-methylenedioxypyrovalerone, and methylone, making possession and sales of products containing these chemical illegal in the United States. This was a 1-year temporary scheduling action, which will enable the Agency to conduct further research regarding the safety of these products, with the possibility that these amines will be listed permanently among others within Schedule I. Although there may be a 6-month delay in the DEA's final decision, it is fully expected that these substances will be on the final controlled substances list, most likely Schedule I. These loopholes in the regulation of these drugs have been exploited by illicit drug manufacturers to incorporate newer drugs or drug classes into these products.[4] In Europe, all 27 members of the European Union (EU) have banned bath salts. There are also two countries outside the EU, Norway and Croatia, that have similar legislation. In the Netherlands, sales or possession is punishable with 6 years in prison or a €45,000 ($56,000) fine.

A number of comprehensive reviews on the patterns of use, pharmacology, and toxicology of bath salts have recently been published.[1,2,5,6] This review focuses on the chemistry, metabolism, and laboratory analysis of synthetic cathinones to fill in gaps on our most recent understanding on how this new class of designer drug and intoxications resulting from their abuse can be handled through the current analytical platforms available in research and clinical laboratories. To set the tone for which cases the laboratory analysis will be used for in bath salts intoxication, however, the review starts with a typical case report and discussion associated with bath salts intoxication that have recently abounded in various medical journals.

CASE REPORT

A 27-year-old woman entered a club with a group of her friends. She had a packet labeled "Cloud 9" in her purse. While in the bathroom, she opened the packet and snorts a white powder. She returned to the dance floor, where a disc jockey was playing loud music. The temperature in the club was very warm and the floor was very crowded. After a few minutes, she became heavily diaphoretic. She sat down for a few minutes but then became tachycardic, restless, and agitated. A few minutes later she suffered a seizure. A medical team attended to her and an ambulance was called; she was then admitted to the emergency room. Her presenting symptoms included headache, palpitations, blood pressure 160/100 mm Hg, temperature 38.5°C, pulse of 105 beats/min. She denied chest pain or any cardiac symptoms and a 12-lead electrocardiogram revealed tachycardia, but was negative for evidence of myocardial ischemia. Her friends told the admitting team that she has a prior medical history of MDMA use but no history of prior hospitalization for use of this or any other drug.

Laboratory results showed hyponatremia (129 mmol/L) and a mild increase in creatine kinase (450 units/L). An arterial blood gas measurement showed no acid–base disturbance and she exhibited good oxygenation. All other results, including renal and liver function tests, were unremarkable. A blood alcohol test was negative. A urine drug screen using immunoassays was ordered, which was negative for cocaine, methamphetamine, MDMA, tetrahydrocannabinol, opiates, and phencyclidine. The patient was treated with intravenous lorazepam as a sedative and to prevent further seizures. The patient was discharged the next day to the care of her parents. A social worker called on the family 72 hours after discharge. The patient complained of blurred vision, moderate depression, and lack of focus and motivation.

Case Discussion

Bath salts use is attractive to young adults largely because of its stimulatory and hallucinogenic properties. The initial effects include an elevation in mood, decreased hostility, and higher empathy. Like other stimulants, this is followed by depression, psychosis, and suicidal ideation. Patients who present to the emergency department with bath salts abuse have a clinical presentation of sympathomimetic stimulation similar to what is observed for cocaine, methamphetamine, and MDMA. The synthetic amines found in bath salts are agonists to α- and β-adrenergic receptors, causing a sustained neuronal released of endogenous norepinephrine, dopamine, and serotonin.[1] There may also be inhibition of reuptake at synaptic junctions. This case exhibited the typical side effects of mephedrone exposure. Although not exhibited in this case, some patients on rarer occasions have experienced more severe toxicities. These include vasospasms that can precipitate to acute myocardial infarction; rhabdomyolysis, which if untreated can lead to renal failure; cyanosis as exhibited by peripheral skin discoloration; and death due to arrhythmias, respiratory distress, and cardiovascular collapse.[7] The agitation can lead to violence against club patrons and emergency department personnel.

CHEMISTRY OF BATH SALTS

Synthetic cathinones are analogues of amphetamines. As a class they are β-keto-phenylisopropylamines, structurally derived from amphetamines by substitution of hydrogen atoms with a carbonyl group at the β-carbon. Hence, most synthetic cathinones have corresponding amphetamines (**Fig. 1**). The presence of the carbonyl group in synthetic cathinones makes these compounds more polar than their corresponding amphetamines. Thus, relative to their amphetamine counterparts, synthetic cathinones have less ability to cross the blood–brain barrier, making them generally less potent in their central nervous system (CNS) effects. Furthermore, the carbonyl group imparts synthetic cathinones with a more planar structure, which may affect their ability to bind different receptors that mediate their psychoactive effects.[1,2]

Like other designer drugs, a large number of compounds comprise synthetic cathinones. The structures of all other members of this class are derived from modifying or adding functional groups around 5 positions in their parent compound cathinone (**Fig. 2**).

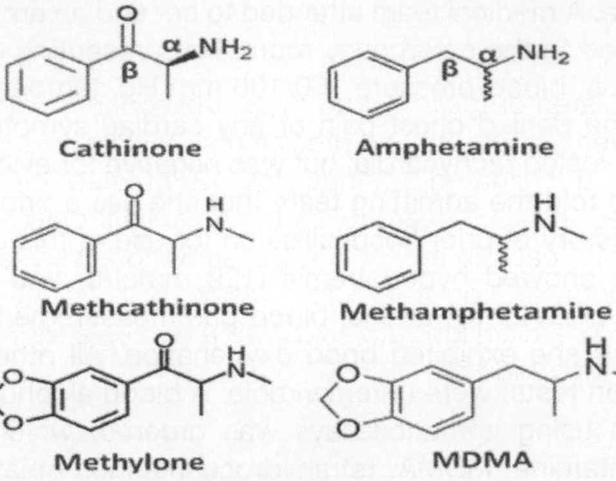

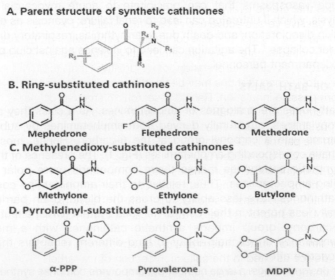

Fig. 1. Cathinones are analogues of amphetamines.

Synthetic cathinones can be grouped according to their pattern of substitution: ring-substituted, methylenedioxy-substituted, and pyrrolidinyl-substituted.

The aromatic ring can be substituted with a wide variety of functional groups in three different positions. The *para* position, however, is a favorite target among illicit drug manufacturers because *para*-substituted phenylisopropylamines exhibit longer half-lives than their *ortho*- and *meta*-substituted isomers and generally have higher potency. Liver enzymes metabolize phenylisopropylamines by hydroxylating the *para* position of the ring[3]; hence, blocking this site via attaching a functional group prolongs metabolism of the resulting compound. The same is thought to be true of synthetic cathinones, although the carbonyl group attached to their ring is a *meta*-directing substituent in electrophilic aromatic substitution. Mephedrone, flephedrone, and methedrone are examples of this group.

A. Parent structure of synthetic cathinones

B. Ring-substituted cathinones

Mephedrone   Flephedrone   Methedrone

C. Methylenedioxy-substituted cathinones

Methylone   Ethylone   Butylone

D. Pyrrolidinyl-substituted cathinones

α-PPP   Pyrovalerone   MDPV

Fig. 2. Synthetic cathinones can be classified into groups according to their patterns of substitution.

Like amphetamines, addition of the methylenedioxy ring to cathinones generates a similar group of compounds with slightly different properties. In amphetamines, addition of this group facilitates the entactogenic effects of MDMA.[5] This may not necessarily be the case for cathinones, but methylenedioxy-substituted cathinones penetrate the blood–brain barrier better and may have more serotonergic effects than other ring-substituted cathinones, as observed for methylone.[7] Ethylone, butylone, and pentylone also belong to this group.

Finally, a unique class of synthetic cathinones has its amino group as part of the pyrrolidine ring. The presence of the pyrrolidine ring in this group imparts it with more lipophilicity, which may allow these cathinones to penetrate the blood–brain barrier better, increasing their potential potency. α-Pyrillidonopropiophenone (α-PPP) and pyrovalerone are examples. Some members of this group also have methylenedioxy rings that make them even more lipophilic, hence more potent. This is true in the case of methylenedioxypyrrolidino- propiophenone (MDPPP), methylenedioxypyrrolidino-butiophenone (MDPBP), and methylenedioxypyrrovalerone (MDPV).

Illicit drug manufacturers have explored each of these groups of synthetic cathinones. With renewed interest in synthetic cathinones beginning in the mid-2000s, mephedrone was the first to gain popularity. When various European countries started to ban this compound, methylone and MDPV started appearing in the market. The synthetic route to produce some of these compounds bears a close resemblance to the production of amphetamines. Methcathinone, for example, can be clandestinely produced starting with pseudoephedrine. Instead of reducing this starting material, as for methamphetamine production, it is oxidized with potassium permanganate in the presence of sulfuric acid.[1] In fact, the Parkinson-like syndrome observed in chronic users of methcathinone in the former Soviet Union in the 1970s and the United States in the 1990s was linked to residual manganese in methcathinone drugs to which users are inadvertently exposed.[8]

METABOLISM

Not much is known about the metabolism of synthetic cathinones. Most of what is known about the metabolism of these compounds is from recent studies on the more popular ingredients of "bath salts" such as mephedrone, fluoromethcathinone, methylone, and MDPV[9–14]; extrapolations from what are known about their corresponding amphetamines and cathinone,[3,15]; and a series of studies conducted by Maurer and colleagues in the early 2000s.[16–22]

Like amphetamines, synthetic cathinones are extensively metabolized in the liver. They undergo both phase I and II reactions. There are four potential sites that phase I metabolic enzymes could modify in cathinone derivatives. Enzyme action on these sites may lead to (1) N-dealkylation of the substituted amino group, (2) reduction of the carbonyl group to alcohol, (3) hydroxylation of the aromatic ring, and (4) demethylenation of the methylenedioxy group (**Fig. 3**). Further reactions may then occur in the initial products of these reactions such as the transfer of a methyl group to a hydroxyl group by enzymes such as catechol-O-methyltransferase (COMT), an enzymatic reaction reminiscent of the MDMA metabolic pathway. Ultimately, products of phase I metabolism are then subjected to conjugation reactions by phase II enzymes adding glucuronide or sulfate to hydroxyl or carboxyl groups.[1,23]

The predominant type of phase I reaction varies from one group of synthetic cathinone to another. Mephedrone, for example, seems to undergo all three phase I transformations described previously. A gas chromatography-mass spectrometry (GC-MS) analysis of urine samples from rats and humans with prior exposure to mephedrone suggested that N-demethylation, reduction of the carbonyl group to

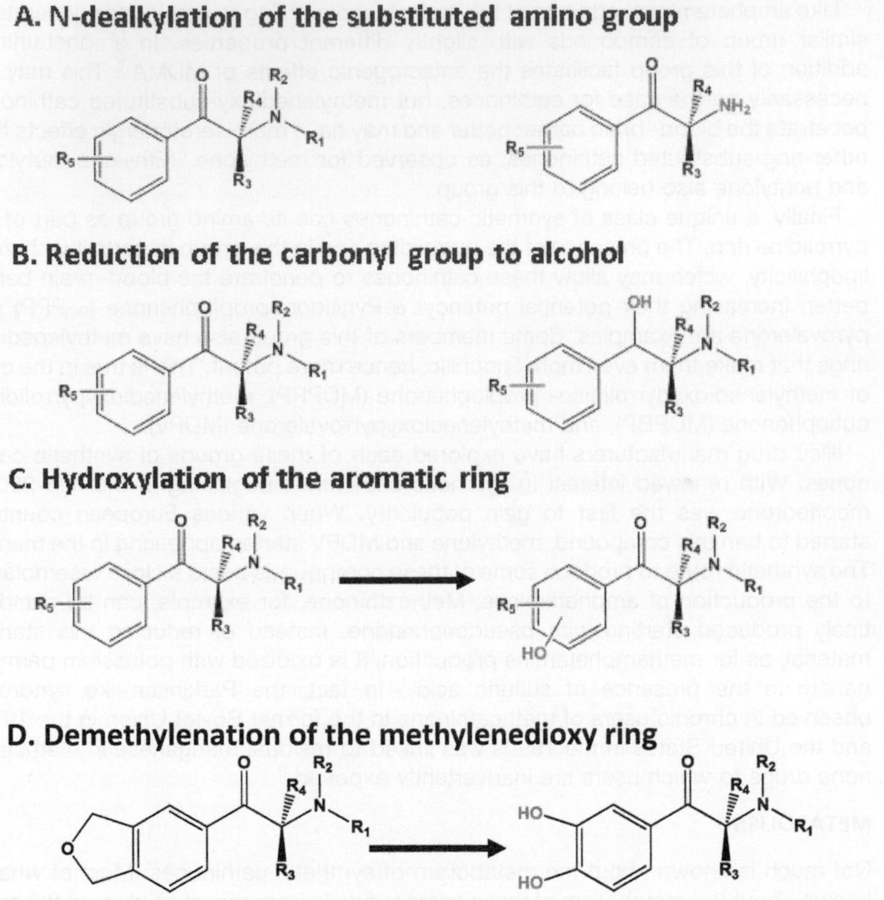

A. N-dealkylation of the substituted amino group

B. Reduction of the carbonyl group to alcohol

C. Hydroxylation of the aromatic ring

D. Demethylenation of the methylenedioxy ring

Fig. 3. Common phase I reactions undergone by synthetic cathinones.

alcohol, and hydroxylation of the tolyl group all occur in rats and humans. Further oxidation of the hydroxylated tolyl group to a carboxylic acid additionally occurs in humans.[9] The study further suggested that glucuronidation and sulfation of these metabolites also occur. The same set of phase I metabolic reactions were observed for 3-bromemethcathinone and 3-fluromethcathinone in rat urine and human liver microsomes in one study,[22] while another study using rabbit liver slices suggested that ring hydroxylation followed by reduction of the carbonyl group to alcohol and N-demethylation followed by reduction of the resulting amine to imine are the main routes of metabolism for 3-fluoromethcathinone.[12] In both mephedrone and halogenated methcathinones, the unchanged parent drugs are also observed in the urine.

The methylenedioxy-substituted cathinones methylone, ethylone, and butylone seem to follow a metabolic pathway similar to that of MDMA. The primary metabolic pathway for this group starts with demethylenation of the methylenedioxy ring followed by O-methylation through COMT. Both 4'-hydroxy-3'-methoxy (4'-OH-3'-MeO) and 3'-hydroxy-4'-methoxy (3'-OH-4'-MeO) are formed. The former is observed as the major metabolite in rat urine but both are partly conjugated with glucuronides and sulfates. N-dealkylation is a minor pathway for these compounds.

Oxidation of the β-keto group does not occur at all for methylone, while it is also a minor pathway for ethylone and butylone.[13,23,24]

Because of its methylenedioxy ring, the pyrrolidinyl-substituted cathinone MDPV is likewise metabolized by demethylation followed by methylation.[10,11] One study showed that indeed catechol pyrovalerone and methylcatechol pyrovalerone are the major metabolites obtained in vitro when MDPV is incubated with human liver microsomes.[11] In another study, however, additional metabolic reactions were postulated to occur in humans including hydroxylation of the propyl side chain and hydroxylation of the pyrrolidine ring, followed by its dehydrogenation to its corresponding lactam and its eventual degradation to primary amine. The corresponding metabolic pathway in rats seems to be more extensive, forming various oxidative products.[10] Glucuronidation and sulfation of some of these phase I metabolites also occur. The closely related MDPPP exhibits the same major metabolic reactions as MDPV.[19]

Oxidation of the pyrrolidine ring and its dehydrogenation to its corresponding lactam seem to be a common pathway for other pyrrolidinyl-substituted cathinones. α-PPP, 4'-methyl-α-pyrrolidinopropiophenone (MPPP), and 4'-methoxy-α-pryyolidinopropiophenone (MOPPP) all undergo this metabolic reaction, along with hydroxylation of the aromatic ring in the 4'-position.[16,18,20] Oxidative deamination or double dealkylation to a primary amine of the pyrrolidine ring also occurs, while reduction of the carbonyl group to a secondary alcohol is a minor pathway.

Consistent with anecdotal accounts of rapid onset and resolution of bath salts effects, initial studies on the pharmacokinetics of synthetic cathinones indicate that these compounds generally have a short half-life. Insufflation (snorting) and oral ingestion are the most common routes of administration of bath salts, although rectal insertion as enema and intramuscular and intravascular injections have also been reported.[24,25] Typical doses for mephedrone and methylone reported by users are 100 to 200 mg orally. Users also report that when mephedrone is taken by insufflation, effects can take effect within 10 to 20 minutes, peak in less than 30 minutes, and rapidly decline within 1 to 2 hours. Onset of effects takes longer with oral ingestion (within 20–40 minutes), and consequently, effects can be felt as long as 4 hours. Combining the routes of administration has also been reported to hasten the onset of effects and maintain them for a longer time.[1,23,26] MPDV seems to be more potent, with doses of 10 to 15 mg typically causing effects within 15 to 30 minutes and lasting 2 to 7 hours.[2]

Animal studies on pyrovalerone in the 1970s indicated that pyrovalerone is both rapidly absorbed in the stomach and excreted in the urine. It is completely absorbed in the stomach in 45 minutes, and about 70% of it is excreted in urine 4 hours after oral ingestion. Intravenous injection allowed detection of 20% of the drug in urine within 20 minutes.[23,27] Even with renewed interest in synthetic cathinones in the last 3 years, no other pharmacokinetic data on any other synthetic cathinones have been reported in the literature.

LABORATORY ANALYSIS

Similar to other designer drugs, urine and serum drug screens are not yet routinely available for synthetic cathinones. Until recently, no immunoassay has been commercially available for synthetic cathinones. One immunoassay kit was recently released in the United Kingdom; however, its clinical utility still awaits evaluation by clinical laboratories. The few studies published on the analysis of synthetic cathinones in bath salts products, urine, blood, gastric contents, and hair employ GC-MS; liquid chromatography-tandem mass spectrometry (LC-MS/MS); liquid chromatography-time-of-flight mass spectrometry (TOF LC-MS); and in a couple of research laboratories, nuclear magnetic resonance (NMR) spectroscopy.[9,28–38]

A few groups have looked at the major drug ingredients of products sold as bath salts. Initial reports involved analysis of single products using high-resolution mass spectrometry (HRMS) and NMR to determine their drug components. The use of NMR is almost imperative for these initial studies because structure elucidation of the unknown drugs is required with the unavailability of commercial reference standards. This is how mephedrone was established to be the major component of the first wave of bath salts products that became popular in Europe. Soon after deaths were reported from bath salts or legal highs in Europe, for instance, Gibbons and Zloh analyzed a legal high product using HRMS, NMR, elemental composition analysis, and polarimetry. The study identified mephedrone to be the major component of a legal high product. They also confirmed that mephedrone is present as a racemic mixture.[35]

Soon after the United Kingdom banned mephedrone and synthetic cathinone analogues in April, 2010, second-generation legal highs swiftly appeared in drug markets. The most prominent of this is "energy-1 or NRG-1," a product that claims to contain naphyrone, a β-keto amphetamine that is not a derivative of cathinone; hence, it is not necessarily covered by the ban. One group analyzed bath salts products marketed after the ban for their drug content. Twenty-four products obtained from 18 U.K.-based Web sites were analyzed using GC-MS, NMR, and comparison with reference standards. Of the 24 products analyzed, only one contained naphyrone. Most of the products still contained synthetic cathinones covered by the ban either alone or in a mixture including mephedrone itself in 25% of the products. Other cathinone derivatives were identified such as MPDV, flephedrone, butylone, and 4-methyl-N-ethylcathinone, indicating a shift in the product makeup of designer drugs. Some products also contain drugs other than synthetic cathinone, such as caffeine, lidocaine, benzocaine, and procaine. Six products contain these drugs alone without any synthetic cathinone.[39] Caffeine, being a stimulant, is not a surprising find. The three other drugs are local anesthetics and are presumably added to produce numbness and deflect the pain associated with snorting the drug. In a follow-up study, three other novel synthetic cathinones were discovered to make up bath salts products including pentylone, MDPBP, and MPPP. One of the products contained four different synthetic cathinones.[40] The ban has sparked what is inevitable for designer drugs such as bath salts: the switch in drug formulation as soon as a legal ban on a popular ingredient is passed.

Aside from synthetic cathinones, other classes of compounds have been incorporated in second-generation legal high or bath salts products. With the ban on all analogues of synthetic cathinones in the United Kingdom, the only way to avoid prosecution for drug manufacturers is to explore substitutes that are not derivatives of cathinone. Naphyrone is one of these drugs but it was also banned in the United Kingdom as of July, 2010.[41] In the latter half of 2010, other drug classes such as aminoindanes and benzofurans found their way into the legal high market. Because there are no legislations banning these compound classes, selling them as legal highs is indeed legal. To test the authenticity of the claims of these products, seven legal high products were tested for their drug composition using Fourier transform infrared (FT-IR) spectroscopy and GC-MS. The components of the drugs obtained are declared as one among methylenedioxyaminoindane (MDAI), 5-iodo-2-aminoindane (5-IAI), and 6-(2-aminopropyl)benzofuran (6-APB). Results of the analysis revealed that only one of the seven products actually contained what was declared in its label; the six other products contained large amounts of caffeine. Interestingly, five of the seven products contained the same mixture of three drugs (benzylpiperazine, 3-trifluoromethylpiperazine, and caffeine), contrary to the drugs declared in each of their labels.[42] It was concluded that manufacturers can just be rebranding the same product and declaring it as some other drug that is not banned yet. Inconsistencies in the actual components of legal high products bearing the same brand name were also observed.

Because the bath salts epidemic did not reach the United States until the latter part of 2010, the first analysis of bath salts products in the United States was not published until May, 2011. Fifteen products obtained from local smoke shops and convenience stores in Kentucky and Oklahoma were analyzed for their drug content via GC-MS. Each of the 15 products contained one or two of three synthetic cathinones, namely MDPV, mephedrone, and methylone. Contrary to what was true in Europe when bath salts first became popular, mephedrone is not the major synthetic cathinone found in the products analyzed. Instead, MPDV and methylone are found in more products.[43] This is understandable considering that by this time in Europe, mephedrone had already been replaced by other synthetic cathinones, particularly MDPV. The findings of this study eventually became the basis for the DEA ban placing only these three synthetic cathinones temporarily as Schedule I drugs.[44] A more recent study analyzed bath salts products pre- and post- federal ban using TOF LC-MS. The drugs identified in bath salts purchased pre-federal ban are MDPV and methylone, consistent with the previous publication. The drugs identified post-federal ban, however, are completely different and include α-PVP, butylone, and 6-APB.[45] Interestingly, in some of the products analyzed, MPPP was also identified as a component of herbal incense in combination with synthetic cannabinoids.

Due to the lack of immunoassay for synthetic cathinones, their analysis in patient samples is currently limited to specialized testing such as GC-MS and LC-MS/MS. Early reports of synthetic cathinone analysis were mostly through case reports. Mephedrone was measured via GC-MS in blood, urine, and hair in four fatalities. The range of mephedrone levels measured in the postmortem blood was 1.2 to 22 μg/mL. Other drugs of abuse were identified along with mephedrone in three of the four cases. The limit of detection for the developed GC-MS method is 200 ng/mL, which is quite high compared to the value for other amphetamines.[28]

The first reports on synthetic cathinone analysis in a large population of patient samples came from Finland. A serum LC-MS/MS assay was developed to assess the incidence of MPDV intoxication among drivers suspected to be under the influence of drugs (DUID). The assay was developed using an electrospray ionization source in positive polarity. MDPV was detected and quantified using two transitions (m/z 276/126 and 276/135) with 3,4-methylenedioxy-N-ethylamphetamine (MDEA)-d5 as internal standard. The limits of detection and quantification for the assay are 3 and 11 ng/mL, respectively, while its linear dynamic range is 10 to 500 ng/mL. MDPV was detected in 259 drivers, which represented about 5.7% of all DUID cases in 1 year. The range of MDPV levels detected is 16 to greater than 8000 ng/mL. Other drugs of abuse were detected together with MDPV. Amphetamine (80%) and benzodiazepine were among the most common drugs detected along with MDPV.[46] A urine assay for MDPV was also developed using GC-MS to monitor MDPV and other amphetamine-like drugs in opioid-dependent patients undergoing opioid substitution treatment. The urine samples were prepared by liquid–liquid extraction with toluene and the resulting extract was derivatized with heptafluorobutyric acid and acid anhydride. MDPV was analyzed using electron ionization GC-MS in selected ion monitoring mode using m/z 276 as target ion along with three abundant fragments as qualifier ions. The assay has limits of detection and quantification of 10 and 20 ng/mL, respectively and a linear dynamic range of 20 to 2000 ng/mL. MDPV was detected in 9 of 34 urines, 4 of which also tested positive for amphetamine.[47]

A multidrug panel for synthetic cathinones and their related ephedrines in live and postmortem blood has also been developed using LC-MS/MS. Nine cathinones and six ephedrines were included in the panel using electrospray ionization as ion source in the positive polarity. Using protein precipitation for sample preparation, the recoveries for analytes in the assay span 87% to 106% in the concentration range of 10 to 250 ng/mL. The limits of detection observed for the analytes were in the range 0.5 to 3 ng/mL. The cathinones were observed to be unstable in whole blood and sample extracts under neutral conditions, but acidification of the sample matrix helped improved their stability.[34] A qualitative urine drug screen for eight compounds found in legal highs has also been developed using ultra performance (UP)LC-MS/MS. Five of the analytes are synthetic cathinones and are detected using two transitions through electrospray ionization in the positive polarity. Urines were prepared by dilute and shoot, and the cutoff for analyte identification was set at 1000 ng/mL to mirror what was set for amphetamine for workplace drug testing.

In the United States, only one large study has been published that measured synthetic cathinones in patients' blood/serum and urine. A quantitative GC-MS method for mephedrone and MDPV was developed in blood/serum and urine to analyze samples collected from cases reported to the Kentucky and Louisiana Poison Control Centers. The authors did not report the method's analytical characteristics but the reported ranges for the calibrators span 25 to 150 ng/mL. MDPV was detected in 13 of 17 patient blood/serum samples (range: 21–241 ng/mL) and three of five urine samples (range: 34–1386 ng/mL). The four blood/serum samples with no synthetic cathinone detected reported last use of bath salts more than 20 hours before presentation. No mephedrone level was reported in the study. Postmortem samples were also analyzed for the single fatality case. MDPV was detected in blood at 170 ng/mL and in urine at 1400 ng/mL.[43]

The authors' laboratory has developed a method for measuring synthetic cathinones using TOF LC-MS. So far, quantitative measurements of synthetic cathinones in bath salts products, serum, and urine were performed on six cases, of which one has been published.[48] In the published case, MDPV, flephedrone, and caffeine were detected in the bath salts product taken by the patient. MDPV was measured in his blood and urine at 186 and 136 ng/mL, respectively. Flephedrone was measured at higher levels in his serum and urine at 346 and 257 ng/mL, respectively. Synthetic cathinones detected in the other cases include MDPV, MDPPP, α-PVP, and pentedrone.

The ever-changing landscape of drugs sold as bath salts poses a tremendous challenge in the development of clinical tests for this class of drugs. Traditional GC-MS or LC-MS/MS may not suffice, for as soon as target analytes for these platforms are incorporated in an assay, illicit bath salts manufacturers have move on to a different set of target compounds. HRMS like TOF or quadrupole (Q)TOF LC-MS and LC-Orbitrap may provide the appropriate analytical platform in developing clinical tests for synthetic cathinones and designer drugs, in general. The ability of these platforms to provide full scan mass spectra with high accurate mass measurements allows assignment of potential formula matches to unknown compounds with high confidence. This allows potential discovery of new drugs that are incorporated to bath salts products and their easy incorporation to the developed assay once reference standards become available. These platforms also allow retrospective analysis of acquired data every time a method is expanded to incorporate newer drugs, which can help trace if the drugs have already been used by previous patients. These capabilities allow flexibility in assay development to respond swiftly to changes in the composition of drugs sold commercially.

REFERENCES

1. Kelly J. Cathinone derivatives: a review of their chemistry, pharmacology and toxicology. Drug Test Anal 2011;3:439–53.

2. Rosenbaum CD, Carreiro SP, Babu KM. Here today, gone, tomorrow. . . and back again? A review of herbal marijuana alternatives (K2, Spice), synthetic cathinones (Bath salts), Kratom, *Salvia divinorum*, methoxetamine and piperazines. J Med Toxicol 2012;8:15–32.

3. Carvalho M, Carmo H, Costa VM, et al. Toxicity of amphetamines: an update. Arch Toxicol 2012. [Epub ahead of print].

4. Fass JA, Fass AD, Garcia AS. Synthetic cathinones (bath salts): legal status and patterns of abuse. Ann Pharmacother 2012;46:436–41.

5. Caroll FI, Lewin AH, Mascarella SW, et al. Designer drugs: a medicinal chemistry perspective. Ann N Y Acad Sci 2012;1248:18–38.

6. Hill S, Thomas S. Clinical toxicology of newer recreational drugs. Clin Toxicol (Phila) 2011;49:705–19.

7. Bejhadj-Tahar H, Sadeg N. Methcathinone: a new postindustrial drug. Forensic Sci Int 2005;197:159.

8. De Bie RM, Gladstone RM, Strafella AP, et al. Manganese-induced Parkinsonism associated with methcathinone (Ephedrone) abuse. Arch Neurol 2007;64(6):886–9.

9. Meyer M, Wilhelm J, Peters FT, et al. Beta-keto amphetamines: studies on the metabolism of the designer drug mephedrone and toxicological detection of mephedrone, butylone, and methylone in urine using gas chromatography-mass spectrometry. Anal Bioanal Chem 2010;397:1225–33.

10. Meyer M, Du P, Schuster F, et al. Studies on the metabolism of the α-pyrrolidinophenone designer drug methylenedioxy-pyrovalerone (MDPV) in rat and human urine and human liver microsomes using GC-MS and LC-high resolution MS and its detectability in urine by GC-MS. J Mass Spectrosc 2010;45:1426–42.

11. Strano-Rossi S, Cadwallader A, de la Torre X, et al. Toxicological determination and in vitro metabolism of the designer drug methylenedioxypyrovalerone (MDPV) by gas chromatography/mass spectrometry and liquid chromatography/quadrupole time-of-flight mass spectrometry. Rapid Commun Mass Spectrom 2010;24:2706–14.

12. Pawlik E, Plässer G, Mahler H, et al. Studies on the phase I metabolism of the new designer drug 3-fluoromethcathinone using rabbit liver slices. Int J Legal Med 2011; 126.231–40.

13. Kamata HT, Shima N, Zaitsu K, et al. Metabolism of the recently encountered designer drug, methylone, in humans and rats. Xenobiotica 2006;36:709–23.

14. Mueller D, Rentsch K. Generation of metabolites by an automated online metabolism method using human liver microsomes with subsequent identification by LC-MS(n), and metabolism of 11 cathinones. Anal Bioanal Chem 2012;402:2141–51.

15. Feyissa A, Kelly J. A review of the pharmacological properties of khat. Prog Neuro-Psychopharmacol Biol Psych 2008;32:147–66.

16. Springer D, Peters FT, Fritschi G, et al. Studies on the metabolism and toxicological detection of the new designer drug 4′-methyl-α-pyrrolidinopropiophenone in urine using gas chromatography-mass spectrometry. J Chromatogr B Analyt Technol Biomed Life Sci 2001;773:25–33.

17. Springer D, Peters FT, Fritschi G, et al. New designer drug 4′-methyl-α-pyrrolidino-hexanophenone: studies on its metabolism and toxicological detection in urine using gas chromatography-mass spectrometry. J Chromatogr B Analyt Technol Biomed Life Sci 2003;789:79–91.

18. Springer D, Fritschi G, Maurer HH. Metabolism and toxicological detection of the new designer drug 4′-methoxy-α-pyrrolidinopropiophenone studied in rat urine using gas chromatography–mass spectrometry. J Chromatogr B Analyt Technol Biomed Life Sci 2003;793:331–42.

19. Springer D, Peters FT, Fritschi G, et al. Metabolism and toxicological detection of the new designer drug 3′,4′-methylenedioxy-α-pyrrolidinopropiophenone studied in rat urine using gas chromatography-mass spectrometry. J Chromatogr B Analyt Technol Biomed Life Sci 2003;793:377–88.

20. Springer D, Fritschi G, Maurer HH. Metabolism of the new designer drug α-pyrrolidinopropiophenone (PPP) and the toxicological detection of 4′-methyl-α-pyrrolidinopropiophenone (MPPP) studied in rat urine using gas chromatography-mass spectrometry. J Chromatogr B Analyt Technol Biomed Life Sci 2003;796:253–66.

21. Sauer C, Peters FT, Haas C, et al. New designer drug α-pyrrolidinovalerophenone (PVP): studies on its metabolism and toxicological detection in rat urine using gas chromatographic/mass spectrometric techniques. J Mass Spectrom 2008;44:952–64.

22. Meyer MR, Vollmar C, Schwaninger AE, et al. New cathinone-derived designer drugs 3-bromomethcathinone and 3-fluoromethcathinone: studies on their metabolism in rat urine and human liver microsomes using GC-MS and their detectability in urine. J Mass Spectrom 2011;47:253–62.

23. Prosser J, Nelson L. The toxicology of bath salts: a review of synthetic cathinones. J Med Tox 2011. [Epub ahead of print].

24. Zaitsu K, Katagi M, Tatsuno M, et al. Recently abused beta-keto derivatives of methylenedioxyphenylalkylamines: a review of their metabolisms and toxicological analysis. Forensic Toxicol 2011;29:73–84.

25. Carhart-Harris RL, King LA, Nutt DJ. A web-based survey on mephedrone. Drug Alcohol Depend 2011;s118:19–22.

26. James D, Adams RD, Spears R, et al. Clinical characteristics of mephedrone toxicity reported to the UK National Poisons Information Service. Emerg Med J 2010;28:686–9.

27. Michaelis W, Russell JH, Schindler O. The metabolism of pyrovalerone hydrochloride. J Med Chem 1970;13:497–503.

28. Torrannce H, Cooper G. The detection of mepherdrone (4-methylmethcathinone) in four fatalities in Scotland. Forensic Sci Int 2010;202:e62–3.

29. Frison G, Gregio M, Zamengo L, et al. Gas chromatography/mass spectrometry determination of mephedrone in drug seizures after derivatization with 2,2,2–trichloroethyl chloroformate. Rapid Commun Mass Spectrom 2011;25:387–90.

30. Maheux C, Copeland C. Characterization of three methcathinone analogs: 4-methyl-methcathinone, methylone and bk-MBDB. DEA Microgram J 2010;7:42–9.

31. Jankovics P, Varadi A, Tolgyesi L, et al. Identification and characterization of the new designer drug 4′-methylcathinone (4-MEC) and elaboration of a novel liquid chromatography-tandem mass spectrometry (LC-MS/MS) screening method for seven different methcathinone analogs. Forensic Sci Int 2011;210:213–20.

32. Bell C, George C, Kicman AT, et al. Development of a rapid LC-MS/MS method for direct urinalysis of designer drugs. Drug Test Anal 2011;3:496–504.

33. Kikura-Hanajiri R, Kawamura M, Saisho K, et al. The disposition into hair of new designer drugs: methylone, MBDB, methcathinone. J Chromatogr B Analyt Technol Biomed Life Sci 2007;855:121–6.

34. Sørenson LK. Determination of cathinones and related ephedrines in forensic whole blood samples by liquid chromatography-electrospray tandem mass spectrometry. J Chromatogr B Analyt Technol Biomed Life Sci 879:727–36.
35. Gibbons S, Zloh M. An analysis of the legal high mephedrone. Bioorg Med Chem Lett 2010;20:4135–9.
36. Power JD, McGlynn P, Clarke K, et al. The analysis of substituted cathinones. Part 1: chemical analysis of 2-, 3-, and 4-methylmethcathinone. Forensic Sci Int 2011;212: 6–12.
37. McDermott SD, Power JD, Kavanagh P, et al. The analysis of substituted cathinones. Part 2: an investigation into the phenylacetone based isomers of 4-methymethcathinone and N-ethylcathinone. Forensic Sci Int 2011;22:120–7.
38. Wood D, Dargan P. Mephedrone (4-methylmethcathinone): what is new in our understanding of its use and toxicity. Prog Neuropsychopharmacol Biol Psychiatry 2008. [Epub ahead of print].
39. Brandt SD, Sumnall HR, Measham F, et al. Analyses of second-generation "legal highs" in the UK: initial findings. Drug Test Anal 2010;2:377–82.
40. Brandt SD, Freeman S, Sumnall HR, et al. Analysis of NRG "legal highs" in the UK: Identification and formation of novel cathinones. Drug Test Anal 2011;3:569–75.
41. De Paoli G, Maskell P, Pounder D. Naphyrone: analytical profile of the new "legal high" substitute for mephedrone. J Forensic Legal Med 2012;18:93.
42. Baron M, Elie M, Elie L. An analysis of legal highs- do they contain what it says on the tin. Drug Test Anal 2011;3:576–81.
43. Spiller HA, Ryan ML, Weston RG, et al. Clinical experience with analytical confirmation of "bath salts" and "legal highs" (synthetic cathinones) in the United States. Clin Toxicol (Phila) 2011;49:499–505.
44. Drug Enforcement Administration. Schedules of controlled substance: temporary placement of synthetic cathinones into Schedule I. Federal Regist 2011;76(204): 65371–5.
45. Shanks KG, Dahn T, Behonick G, et al. Analysis of first and second generation legal highs for synthetic cannabinoids and synthetic stimulants by ultra-preformance liquid chromatography and time-of-flight mass spectrometry. J Anal Toxicol 2012;36:360–71.
46. Kriikku P, Wilhelm L, Schwarz O, et al. New designer drug of abuse: 3,4-methylenedioxypyrovalerone (MDPV). Findings from apprehended drivers in Finland. Forensic Sci Int 2011;210:195–200.
47. Ojanperä IA, Heikman PK, Rasanen IJ. 2011. Urine analysis of 3,4-methylenedioxypyrovalerone in opioid-dependent patients by gas chromatography-mass spectrometry. Ther Drug Monit 2011;33(2):257–63.
48. Thornton SL, Gerona RR, Thomaszwski CA. Psychosis from a bath salt product containing flephedrone and MDPV with serum, urine and product quantification. J Med Toxicol 2012. [Epub ahead of print].

The Utility of Immunoassays for Urine Drug Testing

Stacy E.F. Melanson, MD, PhD

KEYWORDS

- Urine drug testing • Qualitative immunoassays • Method validation
- Cross-reactivity • Point of care testing

KEY POINTS

- Immunoassays, as opposed to chromatographic or mass spectrometry methods, are clinically desirable because they provide a rapid turnaround time, allow physicians to make timely decisions regarding patient management, and are more easily integrated into the laboratory workflow.
- Accuracy and precision studies are required, at a minimum, to validate all US Food and Drug Administration–approved qualitative immunoassays for drugs of abuse.
- Laboratory directors must determine an appropriate sample type, test menu, cutoffs, method of reporting (eg, quantitative vs qualitative), and testing location (eg, central laboratory vs point of care), as well as recognize and reduce analytical interferences and potential sample adulteration.
- Although immunoassays are rapid, relatively inexpensive, and easy to automate, there are some limitations including poor sensitivity and specificity.
- Because of the breadth and complexity of testing, clinicians are frequently unaware of the limitations of urine drug screens and how inaccurate interpretation of results can adversely affect patient management; therefore, laboratory directors play an integral role in interpreting urine drug test results and communicating results to clinicians.

INTRODUCTION

Substance abuse is a significant problem in the United States.[1] Over 2.1 million emergency department visits in 2009 were associated with drug misuse or abuse, of which 47% involved an illicit drug and 31.8% involved alcohol. Cocaine, marijuana, alcohol, and heroin were the most commonly abused drugs. In addition, pain and addiction management physicians are managing an increasing number of patients with prescriptions for addictive and/or narcotic drugs. Consequently, 52.1% of emergency department visits involved inappropriate use of pharmaceutical drugs.

The author has nothing to disclose.
Department of Pathology, Brigham and Women's Hospital, 75 Francis Street, Boston, MA 02115, USA
E-mail address: semelanson@partners.org

Clin Lab Med 32 (2012) 429–447
http://dx.doi.org/10.1016/j.cll.2012.06.004
0272-2712/12/$ – see front matter © 2012 Elsevier Inc. All rights reserved.
labmed.theclinics.com

Because of the extent of drug abuse in the population, urine drug testing (UDT) for drugs of abuse (DOA) is commonly performed in laboratories to assist with patient management.

There are a variety of clinical settings and/or specialties in which UDT is useful for the clinical management of patients: in the emergent setting to evaluate potential drug overdose or drug abuse, in obstetrics to diagnosis and manage pregnant patients who are abusing drugs, in pediatrics to evaluate newborns for in utero drug exposure, in drug dependency programs to ensure abstinence, in psychiatry and addiction medicine to monitor compliance, and in pain management to detect potential drug abuse, undisclosed use, or diversion.[2–5] UDT is common not only in clinical settings but is also performed as part of workplace drug testing programs or for legal and forensic purposes. Although the principles and limitations of immunoassays apply to both clinical and nonclinical settings, this article focuses on the implementation and clinical utility of UDT to evaluate potential drug abuse or overdose primarily in the emergent care setting. For detailed discussion of pain management drug testing, neonatal drug testing, toxicology testing in alternative matrices, and principles of forensic toxicology testing, refer to articles elsewhere in this issue.

UDT, or urine drug screening (UDS), is most commonly performed using qualitative immunoassays. This article discusses the principles of common immunoassays; how to validate qualitative immunoassays; how to decide on appropriate specimen type, test menu, and cutoff; the limitations of utilizing immunoassays; and how to communicate test results to clinicians. Some discussion of UDT at the point of care (POC) is also integrated throughout the article.

PRINCIPLES OF COMMON IMMUNOASSAYS

Immunoassays, as opposed to chromatographic or mass spectrometry methods, are clinically desirable because they provide a rapid turnaround time, allow physicians to make timely decisions regarding patient management, and are more easily integrated into the laboratory workflow. Immunoassays can be performed on automated chemistry analyzers and therefore can provide rapid results 24/7, which is particularly important in the emergent care setting where results are needed immediately to confirm clinical suspicion of overdose or drug abuse.[2,6,7] The analytical performance of immunoassays is also acceptable, and the currently available assays screen well for DOA. Furthermore, immunoassays are cost-effective, because the testing can usually be added to existing automated platforms, and laboratories can rapidly introduce new immunoassays if necessary. However, there are limitations to immunoassays, which will be discussed in a later section.

General Principles

Most DOA in urine are measured using competitive immunoassays. In competitive immunoassays the drug from the patient's specimen competes for binding with a fixed amount of labeled drug. Drugs can be labeled with fluorescent, chemiluminescent, or electrochemiluminescent moieties, or with an enzyme capable of generating colored, fluorescent, or chemiluminescent product. Most currently available methods use assay antibodies attached to microparticles suspended in reaction mixture and are optimized to allow rapid equilibration and short assay times. In addition, most current immunoassays for UDT are homogenous, as opposed to heterogenous, and require no separation from microparticles because the signal generated is different in the bound and unbound states.

The majority of UDT results by immunoassay are reported qualitatively based on a specific cutoff concentration whose signal is defined by the assays' calibrator.

Positive results reflect a concentration above the calibrator cutoff but do not indicate the drug or drugs present or the concentrations. Negative results reflect concentrations below the cutoff and do not exclude the presence of drug or metabolite. Samples close to the cutoff may give negative or positive results depending on the precision of the assay and other sample conditions.

The antibody in immunoassays used for UDT can be designed to detect a specific class of compounds (eg, barbiturates), a parent drug (eg, methadone), or a metabolite (eg, benzoylecgonine, a metabolite of cocaine), and performance can vary based on the assays' characteristics. In assays designed to detect a class of drugs, the antibody specificity varies within the drug class, and each individual drug within the class requires a different urine concentration to trigger a positive result (ie, different than the calibrator used to define the cutoff). Certain antibodies may also cross-react with medications outside the target drug class, leading to false-positive results. Therefore, if definitive identification of the drug and/or quantitative analysis is desired, other methodologies are necessary.[8] These limitations and scenarios in which more specific confirmation testing (eg, liquid chromatography–tandem mass spectrometry [LC-MS/MS] or gas chromatography-mass spectrometry [GC-MS]) would be useful are discussed in a later section.

Specific Immunoassay Principles

Several different automated and POC immunoassay techniques are available including enzyme immunoassay (EIA) (eg, enzyme-multiplied immunoassay technology [EMIT], Siemens Healthcare Diagnostics, Malvern, PA, USA), kinetic interaction of microparticle in solution (KIMS), and cloned enzyme donor immunoassay (CEDIA).

EIA assays are based on competitive binding between enzyme-labeled drugs (ie, active enzyme–drug conjugate) and drug in the patient specimen for drug-specific antibodies (**Fig. 1**). When drug is not present in the patient, the enzyme-labeled drug binds to the antibody and the substrate cannot be cleaved by the enzyme to product (see **Fig. 1**A). The result is no change in absorbance over time. When drug is present in the patient, the enzyme-labeled drug is free to interact with the substrate and produce a product, NADH, which absorbs at 340 nm (see **Fig. 1**B). Increasing amount of drug is proportional to increasing absorbance over time. EIA assays can be used on most automated chemistry analyzers.

The KIMS assay (Roche Diagnostics, Indianapolis, IN, USA) uses an antidrug antibody and a labeled microparticle (ie, microparticle-drug conjugate) (**Fig. 2**).[9] In the absence of drug in the patient, the antibody complexes with the labeled microparticle, forms an aggregate, and leads to an increase in absorbance (see **Fig. 2**A). The presence of drug inhibits aggregate formation resulting in a decrease in absorbance (see **Fig. 2**B).

Microgenics (now Thermo Scientific, Fremont, CA, USA) developed the CEDIA assays, which use recombinant DNA technology (**Fig. 3**).[10] The enzyme beta-galactosidase was engineered into two inactive fragments, the enzyme donor (ED) and the enzyme acceptor (EA). The drug in the specimen competes with the drug conjugated to the ED fragment for antibody binding. In the absence of drug, the ED-antibody conjugate remains intact, preventing the formation of an active enzyme and resulting in no change in absorbance over time (see **Fig. 3**A). In the presence of drug, the ED is free to combine with the EA to form the active enzyme, cleave the substrate, and form a product that absorbs light at 570 nm (see **Fig. 3**B). The amount of drug present in the patient is proportional to the increase in absorbance.

Several POC platforms for DOA testing are available using lateral flow immunochromatography. Lateral low immunochromatography is a competitive immunoassay

A Enzyme Immunoassay: Negative

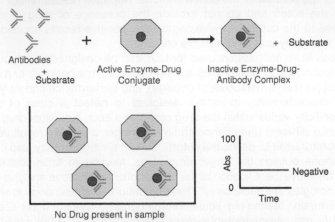

No Drug present in sample

B Enzyme Immunoassay: Positive

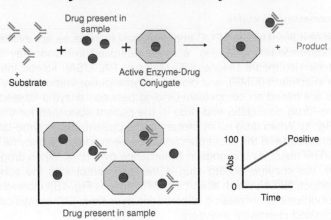

Drug present in sample

Fig. 1. Principle of enzyme immunoassays. (*A*) The reaction associated with a negative result when the patient has no drug in his or her specimen. (*B*) The reaction associated with a positive result when the patient has drug(s) present in his or her specimen.

that is usually read visually to provide qualitative results. Colored latex or colloidal gold microparticles carrying antidrug antibody are mixed with patient's specimen and allowed to flow laterally across a capture zone bearing covalently bound drug. If no drug is present in the specimen, the antidrug antibodies will bind to the capture zone and create a visible line. In the presence of drug, the antibody binds to the drug in the patient and no colored line is produced. Another control zone that binds reagent antibodies is used to confirm proper functioning of the test. A positive result is counterintuitive in most lateral flow immunochromatography assays and indicated by absence of colored line. By contrast, the Biosite Triage POC assay is a fluorescent immunoassay in which the presence of a line indicates a positive response. Furthermore, the results are instrument-read, avoiding interpretative bias. For these reasons the Biosite Triage device and methodology may be preferable to lateral flow immunochromatography.

A   KIMS Technology: Negative

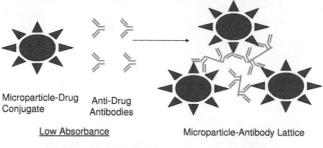

Microparticle-Drug   Anti-Drug
Conjugate   Antibodies

<u>Low Absorbance</u>   Microparticle-Antibody Lattice

<u>High Absorbance</u>

B   KIMS Technology: Positive

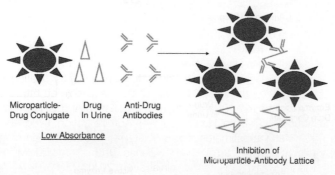

Microparticle-   Drug   Anti-Drug
Drug Conjugate   In Urine   Antibodies

<u>Low Absorbance</u>

Inhibition of
Microparticle-Antibody Lattice

<u>Low Absorbance</u>

Fig. 2. Principle of KIMS. (*A*) The reaction associated with a negative result when the patient has no drug in his or her specimen. (*B*) The reaction associated with a positive result when the patient has drug(s) present in his or her specimen.

METHOD VALIDATION

Accuracy and precision studies are required, at a minimum, for all US Food and Drug Administration (FDA)–approved qualitative immunoassays for DOA. For accuracy studies, it is preferable to compare new immunoassays results with a more sensitive and specific technique such as LC-MS/MS or GC-MS.[11] However, most laboratories do not perform LC-MS/MS or GC-MS. As an alternative, the laboratory validating the test can send validation specimens to its reference laboratory. Reference laboratories will frequently perform the testing for a limited number of specimens free of charge or at a discounted rate. It is also acceptable to compare results to the predicate immunoassay method.

A two-by-two table should be created comparing the results of the reference method (eg, LC-MS/MS, predicate immunoassay) to the test method (ie, new assay). Ideally, at least 100 specimens, including those positive and negative for the drug(s) detected by immunoassay, should be included. It may be challenging to obtain positive specimens. In this case, reference laboratories or colleagues may be able to provide assistance.

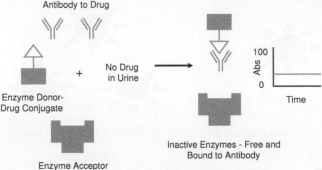

A CEDIA Technology: Negative

B CEDIA Technology: Positive

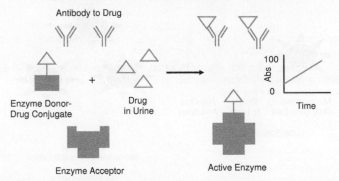

Fig. 3. Principle of CEDIA. (*A*) The reaction associated with a negative result when the patient has no drug in his or her specimen. (*B*) The reaction associated with a positive result when the patient has drug(s) present in his or her specimen.

If the new assay is accurate, the majority of specimens should fall into two categories as depicted in **Table 1**; either negative by both methods (ie, true negative) or positive by both methods (ie, true positive). Scenario A in **Table 1** occurs when the reference method is positive and the test method is negative. This scenario most likely signifies that the test method is falsely negative, especially if the reference method is LC-MS/MS or GC-MS. False-negatives can occur if the test method does not cross-react well with the drug in the patient specimen. If the reference method is the predicate immunoassay, the discrepancy could be due to a false-positive result generated by the reference method. Scenario B occurs when the reference method is

Table 1
Accuracy validation for qualitative immunoassays

	Negative Reference	Positive Reference
Negative Test	True Negative	A
Positive Test	B	True Positive

negative for the drug and test method is positive. This scenario most likely signifies that the test method is falsely positive, especially if the reference method is LC-MS/MS or GC-MS. False-positive results can occur when the test method cross-reacts with a structurally related drug. If the reference method is the predicate immunoassay, the discrepancy could be due to a false-negative result generated by the reference method. Discrepancies (ie, scenario A and B) are expected, but laboratories must determine the cause, particularly in context of the reference method used, and whether or not it is acceptable to implement the testing, considering the discrepancies.

If the new immunoassay is compared with LC-MS/MS or GC-MS, sensitivity and specificity can be calculated using the number of specimens that fall into each category in the two-by-two table, where scenario A is considered false-negative and scenario B is considered false-positive.[11] Sensitivity is [the number of true positives] ÷ [the number of true positives + the number of false negatives]. Specificity is [the number of true negatives] ÷ [the number of true negatives + the number of false positives].

Laboratories also need to conduct precision studies to validate new immunoassays to determine the variability in the results. Precision studies, both within-run and day-to-day, are usually performed using at least two levels of control material, a negative and a positive. However, patient specimens can also be used. A minimum of 20 repeats (over 10 days for day-to-day precision) should be performed for both within-run and day-to-day precision. For qualitative assays it is important that negative control material remain negative (ie, < calibrator cutoff) on repeat testing and that the positive control remain positive (ie, > calibrator cutoff).[11] Laboratories can also use the raw signal provided by the analyzer to calculate a coefficient of variation in the results.[11] Additionally, it can be important examine and document lot-to-lot variability in quality control to determine the variability in different lots of quality control and how that may affect assay performance.[11]

Cross-reactivity and interference studies are important, and the manufacturers of immunoassay kits for UDT usually perform these studies. For FDA-approved tests, laboratories can use these data as part of their test validation. As examples, **Table 2** lists the manufacturer's claims for cross-reactivity of various select benzodiazepines and opiates in the benzodiazepine and opiate assays, respectively. Laboratories should be aware that cross-reactivity for drugs within the class varies widely. Laboratories must also understand that not all drugs and/or their metabolites are tested for cross-reactivity. Similar to cross-reactivity studies, results of interferences studies are outlined by the manufacturers in the package inset.

Although the government and other regulatory agencies are in the process of defining validation requirements for non-FDA approved tests or laboratory-developed tests (LDT), the validation will be more extensive than accuracy and precision. For LDT, cross-reactivity studies should be performed to verify cross-reactivity with not only the drug(s) the immunoassay is designed to detect, but also the metabolites and other classes of drugs.[12] Drug mixes can be purchased from commercial vendors to test cross-reactivity of other classes of drugs. Interference studies with common substances and/or conditions found in the urine (eg, glucose, red blood cells, extremes of pH) should also be performed.[11] The full extent of the validation required for LDT remains to be seen.

IMPLEMENTATION DECISION

Many decisions need to be made before implementing UDT; most are dependent on the clinical setting (eg, emergent care setting vs compliance monitoring) in which the

Table 2
Manufacturer cross-reactivity claims for benzodiazepine and opiate assays

Compound	EIA/EMIT	KIMS	CEDIA
Benzodiazepine Assays			
α-OH-alprazolam	NA	101	163
Alprazolam	91	74	138
Chlordiazepoxide	1330	221	2083
Clonazepam	255	178	188
Diazepam	98	79	110
Lorazepam-glucuronide	>10,000	NA	10,000
Nordiazepam	NA	NA	150
Oxazepam-glucuronide	3600	NA	10,000
Temazepam	138	NA	175
Opiate Assays			
Morphine	300	300	300
Codeine	247	224	240
Hydromorphone	498	1425	526
Hydrocodone	364	1086	625
Oxycodone	5388	>75,000	10,000
Oxymorphone	>20,000	NA	20,000
Morphine-3-glucuronide	626	552	375
Morphine-6-glucuronide	NA	NA	638
6-AM	1088	386	NA

Concentrations in the table are ng/mL required to trigger a positive result.
Abbreviations: 6-AM, 6-acetylmorphine; NA, not available.

test will be used. Laboratory directors must determine an appropriate sample type, test menu, cutoffs, method of reporting (eg, quantitative vs qualitative), and testing location (eg, central laboratory vs POC), as well as recognize and reduce analytical interferences and potential sample adulteration. The policy for reflex testing (ie, when should more specific confirmatory testing be performed) also needs to be established.

Specimen Type

Urine is the specimen of choice for DOA testing in most clinical settings. It is easy to collect and requires no preanalytical preparation. Analytes are relatively concentrated in urine, making urine better than blood for detecting drugs over a longer period time and for assessing compliance and undisclosed use. However, urine can be adulterated, and laboratories should incorporate testing to detect adulteration if it is appropriate for the clinical setting (see article on pain management drug testing elsewhere in this issue).

Unlike blood, urine contains primarily drug metabolites; therefore, results are not reflective of a patient's acute presentation. Furthermore, the concentrations of drug and/or metabolites in the urine are patient-dependent and vary with patient metabolism, hydration status, and renal function. For these reasons, urine concentrations should not be used to predict acute exposure or timing and dose of drug ingestion. Serum should be used to measure analytes (eg, acetaminophen, alcohol, salicylate) in which concentrations reflecting acute exposure are necessary for patient management.

DOA testing in alternative matrices such as meconium, hair, and oral fluid also play an important role in clinical management. These topics are discussed elsewhere in this issue in the articles on toxicology testing in alternative specimen matrices and neonatal drug testing.

Test Menu and Cutoffs

The National Academy of Clinical Biochemistry published guidelines in 2003 for serum and urine drug testing that should be performed by laboratories to accommodate the emergent care setting.[5] According to the guidelines, stat (ie, turnaround time <1 hour with exception of methyl alcohol and ethylene glycol) quantitative serum toxicology testing should include acetaminophen, salicylate, phenobarbital (if urine barbiturates are positive), ethyl alcohol, methyl alcohol, and ethylene glycol. Stat qualitative urine toxicology should include cocaine, opiates, barbiturates, amphetamines, propoxyphene, phencyclidine, and tricyclic antidepressants. However, these recommendations need to be adapted for each laboratory depending on its patient population.

In the emergent care setting, a laboratories test menu should include common illicit drugs in that population in order to confirm clinical suspicion of overdose or drug abuse. The laboratory in collaboration with the clinicians should determine what drugs are commonly abused in their patient population and avoid screening for drugs simply because an assay is offered by the manufacturer of their automated analyzer(s). Furthermore, there should ideally be a clinical intervention for the drugs included in the test menu. For example, a positive result may support the decision and/or prompt a clinician to administer an antidote such as naloxone for opiate overdose. The required turnaround time, test performance, and financial impact of testing should also be considered. As examples, it may not be cost-effective to perform low-volume testing onsite, there may be no commercial assay for some drugs, or the methodology to measure certain drugs may be too sophisticated to maintain and operate. **Table 3** outlines the test menu, methodology, and cutoffs for stat UDT at Brigham and Women's Hospital.

The test menu for compliance monitoring is generally more comprehensive than the emergent care setting in order to detect undisclosed or illicit drug use (see article elsewhere in this issue on pain management drug testing). For example, synthetic opioids such as buprenorphine and fentanyl are frequently prescribed for chronic pain; however, opiate immunoassays, which are designed to detect illicit opiates such

Table 3		
Urine drug testing menu at Brigham and Women's Hospital		
Urine Immunoassay Screen	**Methodology**	**Screen Cutoff (ng/mL)**
Amphetamines	KIMS	1000
Barbiturates	KIMS	200
Benzodiazepines	KIMS	100
Cannabinoids	KIMS	50
Cocaine Metabolite	KIMS	150
Methadone	KIMS	300
Opiates	KIMS	300
Oxycodone	DRI	300

Abbreviation: DRI, Diagnostic Reagents Incorporated.

as heroin, do not detect synthetic opioids. Therefore, immunoassay screens for synthetic opioids, in addition to opiate immunoassays, should be included in the test menu to assess both compliance and illicit use.

The assay cutoff for a specific drug and/or drug classes will depend on the purpose of screening. Of note, laboratories will be limited by the cutoffs provided by the manufacturer for FDA-approved assays. In the emergent care setting it is most important to detect drug toxicity (ie, higher concentrations of drugs) to support clinical suspicion of overdose or to detect drug abuse. For compliance monitoring, cutoffs should be lower in order to detect remote undisclosed or illicit drug use (ie, lower concentrations of drugs).

Method of Reporting/Reflex Testing Algorithms

Results can be reported qualitatively or quantitatively. Quantitative testing is required if a concentration is necessary to guide management, which most frequently applies to drugs measured in the serum. For example, a salicylate concentration, as opposed to a positive or negative result, is necessary to determine how and when to manage a patient with potential salicylate overdose. Quantitative results may also be needed if it is important to follow the concentration over time or correlate the concentration with the dosage ingested as is the case with acetaminophen toxicity. However, in most cases of DOA testing, qualitative results are sufficient to guide patient management.

In certain clinical settings, qualitative results may need to be followed by quantitative testing and/or a more specific assay (eg, LC-MS/MS or GC-MS). For example, a positive opiate screen could be due to heroin use or several different prescription drugs (eg, morphine). If it is important clinically to confirm which drug triggered the positive result and the turnaround time for confirmation testing is acceptable, LC-MS/MS or GC-MS should be performed. Reflex protocols can be implemented by the laboratory or performed on request if warranted by the clinical scenario. Of note, reflex testing algorithms may not be feasible in the emergent care setting because of the relatively prolonged turnaround time.

Location of Testing

Testing can be performed in the central laboratory or at the POC. **Table 4** lists some of the advantages and disadvantages of point-of-care testing (POCT). The performance of point-of-care tests to screen for drugs of abuse is generally comparable with the performance of automated immunoassays. However, performance is assay-dependent and has been studied less extensively in the nonemergent settings. Decentralizing the testing can also decompress the burden on the central laboratory. Furthermore, POCT usually provides a faster turnaround time by providing results at the patient's bedside or during the patient's visit. This turnaround allows clinicians to take immediate clinical action and/or immediately discuss results with patients and make timely decisions regarding patient compliance and prescription renewals. POCT has several disadvantages: it is more expensive than automated testing, the test menu is not as extensive, results are usually more difficult to interpret than automated assays, and regulatory challenges exist. Providers should understand the advantages and disadvantages of POCT and work with the laboratory to ensure accurate and properly documented results if POCT is chosen as a platform for UDT.

Prior to implementation of the testing at the POC, laboratories should work with the clinicians to determine if changes in workflow and improved laboratory turnaround time may obviate the need for POCT and to ensure that POCT will positively impact patient management. If the institution and the laboratory decide to support testing at the POC, there are several helpful tips summarized by Ford.[13] Organizations should

Table 4 Advantages and disadvantages of DOA testing at the POC	
Advantages of POCT	Disadvantages of POCT
Improved turnaround time.	Introduces another platform of testing with different cutoffs and interferences.
Results for many POC tests for DOA are comparable with the central laboratory.	More limited test menu.
Decompresses the central laboratory.	Kits are more expensive, although this expense may be offset by clinical benefits.
Allows clinicians to make more timely decisions, particularly regarding patient compliance.	Subjective result interpretation.
Patients can be more easily observed providing the specimen in the POC setting.	Testing may be performed by nonlaboratorians; therefore, it may be difficult to integrate into workflow and/or maintain compliance. Can be challenging to ensure results are recorded in patient's medical record.

Abbreviation: POCT, point-of-care testing.

attempt to stick to one vendor or one type of device if possible to minimize the extent and length of training and to reduce the number of validations. In addition, the number of staff performing the testing should be minimized so that the staff selected to perform the testing have a high enough test volume and experience to maintain competency. Regardless of who performs the testing, laboratories should be involved in assay selection and validation including pre- and postanalytical variables, in developing standardized training checklists, in educating clinicians regarding the limitations of testing, and in auditing compliance.

When making decisions regarding specimen type, test menu and cutoffs, method of reporting, testing location, and appropriate reflex algorithms, laboratories should work closely with their clinical colleagues. The purpose of screening, the patient population, and standard practice guidelines are particularly important factors to consider.

LIMITATIONS OF URINE IMMUNOASSAYS

Although immunoassays are rapid, relatively inexpensive, and easy to automate, there are some limitations including poor sensitivity and specificity. Results are usually qualitative (ie, positive and negative results are generated), and consequently drug concentrations are not provided. In addition, many immunoassays are class-specific. Therefore, results cannot be attributed to a particular drug or drug metabolite (eg, one cannot determine if a positive result by opiate immunoassay is due to morphine or hydromorphone), and results cannot be used to determine which drug a patient is taking. These limitations may make it difficult to interpret immunoassays.

Specificity

Some immunoassays lack specificity and cross-react with structurally related drugs that are different from the drug or class of drugs that the assay is designed to detect. Therefore, false-positive results are produced (ie, positive by immunoassay screen and negative by confirmation) (Table 5).[14] Some proposed mechanisms of interference include (1) a similarly structured drug or metabolite binds to the antibody, (2) a

Table 5
Immunoassay screens: common causes of false-positives and false-negatives and approximate duration of positive results

Immunoassay Screen	Commonly Detects[a]	Generally Poor Cross-Reactivity (false-negatives)[a]	Common Causes of False-Positives[a]	Approximate Duration of Positive Results in Urine
6-Acetylmorphine (heroin metabolite)	6-acetyl-morphine, Heroin	NA	Morphine[15], Codeine, Methadone	2 to 8 hours after heroin exposure
Amphetamine	d-Amphetamine, d-Methamphetamine, MDMA[b], MDA[b]	l-Amphetamine, l-Methamphetamine, Pseudoephedrine[c], Phentermine, ephedrine	Ranitidine, Chlorpromazine, Others[16-30]	1 to 3 days after use
Barbiturates	Amobarbital, Butalbital, Pentobarbital, Phenobarbital, Secobarbital	Varies significantly by assay	NA	2 to 20 days after use, depending on half-life of drug
Benzodiazepines	Diazepam, Nordiazepam, Oxazepam, Temazepam	Alprazolam, Clonazepam, Lorazepam	Oxaprozin	2 to 14 days after use, depending on half-life of the agent
Buprenorphine	Buprenorphine, Norbuprenorphine	NA	Opiates[12]	2 to 4 days after use

Cannabinoids	▲9-carboxy-THC metabolites	NA	Marinol Niflumic acid	2 to 7 days or more after use (up to 1 month in chronic users)
Cocaine Metabolite	Benzoylecgonine	Cocaine Ecgonine Cocaethylene Ecgonine methyl ester	NA	2 to 3 days after use (> chronic use)
Fentanyl	Fentanyl Despropionyl fentanyl	Norfentanyl Opiates Trazodone	NA	1 to 2 days after use
Methadone	EDDP		NA	3 to 10 days after use
Opiates	Morphine Codeine Hydrocodone Hydromorphone	Oxycodone Oxymorphone	Levofloxacin Ofloxacin	2 to 4 days after use

Abbreviations: EDDP, 2-Ethylidene-1,5-Dimethyl-3,3-Diphenylpyrrolidine; MDA, methylenedioxyamphetamine; MDMA, methylenedioxymethamphetamine; NA, not applicable or unknown; THC, tetrahydrocannabinol.

[a] Cross-reactivities are vendor-specific, and the cross-reactivity varies significantly between vendors. The drugs listed are only examples and do not apply to all immunoassays. Each laboratory should consult their manufacturer's package insert or internal data, if available, for the cross-reactivity and causes of false-positives with their assay

[b] Many amphetamine assays do not cross-react well with MDMA and/or MDA.

[c] Pseudoephedrine, a sympathomimetic amine as opposed as to an illicit amine, from over-the-counter cold medications is a common cause of positive amphetamine immunoassay screens.

drug interferes with the enzyme reaction, (3) a drug produces an erroneous absorbance reading, and (4) a drug leads to secretion of endogenous substances that inhibit antibody binding, interfere with the enzyme reaction, or produce an erroneous absorbance reading.[6,31]

See **Table 5** for a list of some common causes of false-positive results. Therapeutic doses of oxaprozin (Daypro) and levofloxacin can produce false-positive results on benzodiazepines and opiate screens, respectively. In addition, previous studies have shown that false-positive results can be obtained with Microgenics (now Thermo Scientific, Fremont, CA) CEDIA buprenorphine and 6-acetylmorphine (6-AM) assay due to nonspecific antibody cross-reactivity with other opioids including codeine, methadone, morphine, and tramadol.[15] Importantly, many false-positive results have been reported with various amphetamine assays.[16–30]

True positive, but misleading, results may also be obtained with immunoassays. For example, poppy seed ingestion can trigger a positive result on opiate assays because of the presence of morphine. In addition, over-the-counter cold medication containing pseudoephedrine, a sympathomimetic amine, can produce positive amphetamine results.

Sensitivity/Cross-Reactivity

False-negative immunoassay results can be obtained for several reasons: the drug is present below the cutoff, the specific drug is not detected by the immunoassay screen (ie, has low cross-reactivity), or the drug was taken too remotely. **Table 5** denotes the drugs that have relatively poor cross-reactivity in many immunoassay screens. However, cross-reactivity is vendor-specific. The drugs listed in **Table 5** are only examples and do not apply to all immunoassays. Each laboratory should consult its manufacturer's package insert for cross-reactivity data.

Table 6 summarizes data from the College of American Pathologists Urine Drug Screening Proficiency Testing Surveys and compares the results of many laboratories challenged with the same concentration of oxycodone.[32] The data show that oxycodone has variable cross-reactivity in opiate immunoassays. When challenged

Table 6
Percentage of laboratories reporting positive results for oxycodone using opiate immunoassays

Immunoassay Technique	Laboratories Reporting Positive Result for 7500 ng/mL Oxycodone Using Opiate Immunoassay (%)[a]
CEDIA	29
CMI (Triage)	10
EIA (DRI)	NA
EIA (EMIT)	54
FIA	0
FPIA	2
MIA (KIMS)	7

Abbreviations: CMI, colloidal metal immunoassay; DRI, Diagnostic Reagents, Inc; EIA, enzyme immunoassay; FIA, fluorescence immunoassay; FPIA, fluorescence polarization immunoassay; MIA, microparticle immunoassay; NA, not available.

[a] *Data from* College of American Pathologists Urine Drug Testing Proficiency Surveys; and *Adapted from* Melanson SE, Baskin L, Magnani B et al. Interpretation and utility of drug of abuse immunoassays: lessons from laboratory drug testing surveys. Arch Pathol Lab Med 2010;134:735–9.

with 7500 ng/mL of oxycodone, only 0% to 54% of laboratories reported positive results. In other words, negative screening results may be obtained in specimens from patients taking oxycodone when opiate immunoassays are used.[32] Therefore, many laboratories that have a large population of patients prescribed and/or abusing oxycodone or who do not automatically perform an opioid confirmation that detects oxycodone may want to implement an oxycodone-specific immunoassay.

Many benzodiazepine immunoassays have low cross-reactivity for newer benzodiazepine drugs such as lorazepam or clonazepam, in part because the assays do not detect the primary metabolite in urine (eg, lorazepam glucuronide) (see **Tables 2** and **5**). As a result, specimens from patients taking therapeutic or even toxic levels of these drugs may have negative results. There is a high-sensitivity benzodiazepine assay available, which increases detection of lorazepam in the urine by using beta-glucuronidase and cleaving lorazepam glucuronide to lorazepam; however, this assay can still produce false-negative results.

Table 7 further illustrates the variable cross-reactivity of immunoassays by outlining the relative cross-reactivity of various sympathomimetics in select amphetamine immunoassays. Although most assays detect d-amphetamine and d-methamphetamine (ie, cross-reactivity moderate to high), methylenedioxymethamphetamine

Table 7
Relative cross-reactivity of various sympathomimetic compounds using select platforms at 1000 ng/mL cutoff

Compound	EMIT-MAM Emit II Plus (monoclonal)	FPIA Amph/mAMP	CEDIA Amph/Ecstasy	Triage FIA mAMP (monoclonal)
d-Amphetamine	High	High[a]	High[a]	NA
d-Methamphetamine	High[a]	Moderate	NA	High[a]
d,l-Amphetamine	High	Moderate	High	NA
d,l-Methamphetamine	High	Low	High	NA
l-Amphetamine	Moderate	Low	Low	NA
l-Methamphetamine	Moderate	Low	Moderate	Low
MDA	Moderate	Low	High	NA
MDMA	Moderate	Low	High	High
MDEA	Low	NA	High	Moderate
PPA	Low	NA	Low	NA
l-Ephedrine	Low	NA	Low	NA
Pseudoephedrine	Low	NA	Low	NA
Phenteramine	Moderate	Low	Low	NA
Phenmetrazine	Moderate	Low	NA	NA
Methylphenidate	Low	NA	NA	NA
Tyramine	Low	Low	NA	NA

High, cross-reactivity > 50%; Moderate, cross-reactivity 10%–50%; Low, cross-reactivity < 10%.
Abbreviations: Amph, amphetamine; EMIT-MAM, EMIT II Plus monoclonal amphetamine/methamphetamine assay; mAMP, methamphetamine; MDEA, methylenedioxymethamphetamine; NA, not available; PPA, phenylpropanolamine.
 [a] Indicates calibrator.
Data from Snyder ML, Melanson SE. Amphetamines. In: Magnani B, Bissell MG, Kwong TC, et al, editors. Clinical toxicology testing: a guide for laboratory professionals. Northfield (IL): CAP Press; 2012.

(MDMA; ie, Ecstasy) or over-the-counter amphetamine derivatives may not be detected. The urine of a patient abusing MDMA should be positive for amphetamines using the Triage or CEDIA assay (see **Table 7**). However, positive results are less likely to be obtained with the EMIT-II plus monoclonal amphetamine/methamphetamine assay (EMIT-MAM) or fluorescence polarization immunoassay (FPIA) assay. Laboratories that use amphetamine immunoassays that do not detect or have low cross-reactivity for MDMA may consider implementing an MDMA-specific assay depending on its patient population. Furthermore, phentermine has moderate cross-reactivity in the EMIT-MAM assay but low cross-reactivity in the other assays. The l-methamphetamine in Vicks Inhaler may produce a positive result in the EMIT-MAM and CEDIA assays (see **Table 7**). The amphetamine class contains several closely related compounds, some of which need to be detected and others which do not. The final antibody is a compromise, and it is unlikely to be specific for only the desired drugs.[7] Laboratories should choose an amphetamine assay that has the most appropriate cross-reactivity profile for its patient population.

With some urine immunoassays the manufacturer's cross-reactivity claims are not consistent with the performance of the assays. This discrepancy may be due to lot-to-lot variability, differences in population, or the fact that not all compounds and/or metabolites are tested for cross-reactivity. The cross-reactivity claims stated by the manufacturer are only estimates, and the claims should be verified by the laboratory using its patient population if results are in question.

Detection Window

How long a urine specimen remains positive after drug ingestion depends on many factors including dosage, the drug half-life, and a patients' metabolism. Long-acting barbiturates can remain at levels above the cutoff for several weeks after ingestion. Cannabinoids are very lipophilic, and chronic users of cannabinoids will have positive urine specimens for as long as 1 month after use. However, shorter acting drugs such as 6-AM and cocaine are only detectable to several days, and results may be below the cutoff if the window of detection has lapsed. Therefore, the duration of positive results for the drug should be considered when interpreting both negative and positive results (see **Table 5**).

Testing Algorithm/Need for Confirmation

It would be ideal to bypass immunoassay screens and perform a more sensitive and specific confirmatory test (eg, GC-MS, LC-MS/MS) on all specimens to avoid the limitations of immunoassays. However, it is difficult for many laboratories to provide acceptable turnaround time, especially when many laboratories do not have the equipment, expertise, and/or personnel to perform confirmations onsite and must send this testing to a reference laboratory. As a result, most laboratories perform immunoassay screens and alternatively assist clinicians with result interpretation. If appropriate, the laboratory can also automatically reflex to confirmation. The protocol for screening and confirmation will differ between laboratories depending on clinical needs, test menu, methodology used, and testing capability of the laboratory.

RESULT REPORTING AND INTERPRETATION

Because of the breadth and complexity of testing, clinicians are frequently unaware of the limitations of urine drug screens and how inaccurate interpretation of results can adversely affect patient management; therefore, laboratory directors play an integral role in interpreting UDT results and communicating results to clinicians. If

Table 8
Examples of interpretative comments/educational resources for clinicians
General Comments Attached to Results
1. Screening test, confirmation required if definitive result is needed.
2. Consult the laboratory (insert contact name and number) for patient specific toxicology interpretation.
3. Negative results do not exclude the presence of the drug.
Test-Specific Interpretative Footnotes
4. Oxaprozin may cause a false positive benzodiazepine screening result.
5. Negative results may be obtained in patients taking therapeutic or supratherapeutic doses of lorazepam.
Informational Guidelines
6. Test-specific comments printed on the laboratory requisition or informational handout.
7. Development of an intranet site describing test panel, methodology, limitations, and recommendations for follow-up testing.

results are interpreted incorrectly, it can have both clinical and medicolegal consequences for the patient.

Table 8 lists some examples of how laboratories can assist with interpretation. General comments can be attached to results (comments 1–3, **Table 8**). Foremost, clinicians should be made aware who to contact in the laboratory with questions (comment 2, **Table 8**). Results can be reported as presumptive positive, or negative according to a defined cutoff value (comment 1, **Table 8**). It can be clarified that presumptive positive results only indicate the presence of the drug or metabolite in urine and do not indicate or measure intoxication or efficacy of elimination. Furthermore, it can be stated that negative results reflect concentrations that fall below the cutoff and do not necessarily exclude the presence of the drug or metabolite (comment 3, **Table 8**). Clinicians should also understand that confirmation testing is not routinely performed in UDS (comment 1, **Table 8**). In addition, for confirmation of a positive result or further testing on a negative result, the urine should be assayed by an alternative method, which may take several days when sent to reference laboratory.

Comments may also be attached to a specific test to indicate common causes of false-positive or negative results (comments 4-5, **Table 8**). The laboratory can also provide clinicians with electronic resources tailored to common questions posed by clinicians. This provision can be accomplished by informational handouts or an internal Web site specific to that laboratory (comments 6-7, **Table 8**). Laboratories should work with clinicians to institute comments and resources with the greatest clinical impact.

ACKNOWLEDGMENTS

The author would like to acknowledge Marion Snyder for her important contributions to the content and figures in this article.

REFERENCES

1. Substance Abuse and Mental Health Services Administration. Data, outcomes, and quality. Available at: www.samhsa.gov/data/DAWN.aspx. Accessed April 10, 2012.
2. Hammett-Stabler CA, Pesce AJ, Cannon DJ. Urine drug screening in the medical setting. Clin Chim Acta 2002;315:125–35.

3. Heit HA, Gourlay DL. Urine drug testing in pain medicine. J Pain Symptom Manage 2004;27:260–7.
4. Trescot AM, Boswell MV, Atluri SL, et al. Opioid guidelines in the management of chronic non-cancer pain. Pain Physician 2006;9:1–39.
5. Wu AH, McKay C, Broussard LA, et al. National academy of clinical biochemistry laboratory medicine practice guidelines: recommendations for the use of laboratory tests to support poisoned patients who present to the emergency department. Clin Chem 2003;49:357–79.
6. Colbert DL. Drug abuse screening with immunoassays: unexpected cross-reactivities and other pitfalls. Br J Biomed Sci 1994;5:136–46.
7. Melanson SE, Magnani B. False positive urine drug screens: what clinicians should know and when the laboratory should be consulted? News Path 2006:1–3.
8. Rainey PM, Baird GS. Analytical methodologies for the toxicology laboratory. In: Magnani BBissell MGKwong TC, et al. editors.Clinical toxicology testing: a guide for laboratory professionals. Northfield (IL): CAP Press; 2012. p. 83–96.
9. Lu NT, Taylor BG. Drug screening and confirmation by GC-MS: comparison of EMIT II and Online KIMS against 10 drugs between US and England laboratories. Forensic Sci Int 2006;157:106–16.
10. Armbruster DA, Hubster EC, Kaufman MS, et al. Cloned enzyme donor immunoassay (CEDIA) for drugs-of-abuse screening. Clin Chem 1995;41:92–8.
11. Snyder ML, Jarolim P, Melanson SE. A new automated urine fentanyl immunoassay: technical performance and clinical utility for monitoring fentanyl compliance. Clin Chim Acta 2011;412:946–51.
12. Melanson SE, Snyder ML, Jarolim P, et al. A new highly specific buprenorphine immunoassay for monitoring buprenorphine compliance and abuse. J Anal Toxicol 2012;36:201–6.
13. Ford A. Eye the basics, not baubles, for point-of-care testing. CAP Today 2010.
14. Brahm NC, Yeager LL, Fox MD, et al. Commonly prescribed medications and potential false-positive urine drug screens. Am J Health Syst Pharm 2010;67:1344–50.
15. Pavlic M, Libiseller K, Grubwieser P, et al. Cross-reactivity of the CEDIA buprenorphine assay with opiates: an Austrian phenomenon? Int J Legal Med 2005;119:378–81.
16. Badcock NR, Zoanetti GD. Benzathine interference in the EMIT-st urine amphetamine assay. Clin Chem 1987;33:1080.
17. Crane T, Badminton MN, Dawson CM, et al. Mefenamic acid prevents assessment of drug abuse with EMIT assays. Clin Chem 1993;39:549.
18. Grinstead GF. Ranitidine and high concentrations of phenylpropanolamine cross react in the EMIT monoclonal amphetamine/methamphetamine assay. Clin Chem 1989;35:1998–9.
19. Jones R, Klette K, Kuhlman JJ, et al. Trimethobenzamide cross-reacts in immunoassays of amphetamine/methamphetamine. Clin Chem 1993;39:699–700.
20. Kelly KL. Ranitidine cross-reactivity in the EMIT d.a.u. Monoclonal Amphetamine/ Methamphetamine Assay. Clin Chem 1990;36:1391–2.
21. Melanson SE, Lee-Lewandrowski E, Griggs DA, et al. Reduced interference by phenothiazines in amphetamine drug of abuse immunoassays. Arch Pathol Lab Med 2006;130:1834–8.
22. Merigian KS, Browning R, Kellerman A. Doxepin causing false-positive urine test for amphetamine. Ann Emerg Med 1993;22:1370.
23. Merigian KS, Browning RG. Desipramine and amantadine causing false-positive urine test for amphetamine. Ann Emerg Med 1993;22:1927–8.
24. Nixon AL, Long WH, Puopolo PR, et al. Bupropion metabolites produce false-positive urine amphetamine results. Clin Chem 1995;41:955–6.

25. Olsen KM, Gulliksen M, Christophersen AS. Metabolites of chlorpromazine and brompheniramine may cause false-positive urine amphetamine results with monoclonal EMIT d.a.u. immunoassay. Clin Chem 1992;38:611–2.

26. Papa P, Rocchi L, Mainardi C, et al. Buflomedil interference with the monoclonal EMIT d.a.u. amphetamine/methamphetamine immunoassay. Eur J Clin Chem Clin Biochem 1997;35:369–70.

27. Poklis A, Hall KV, Still J, et al. Ranitidine interference with the monoclonal EMIT d.a.u. amphetamine/methamphetamine immunoassay. J Anal Toxicol 1991;15:101–3.

28. Roberge RJ, Luellen JR, Reed S. False-positive amphetamine screen following a trazodone overdose. J Toxicol Clin Toxicol 2001;39:181–2.

29. Schmolke M, Hallbach J, Guder WG. False-positive results for urine amphetamine and opiate immunoassays in a patient intoxicated with perazine. Clin Chem 1996;42:1725–6.

30. Smith-Kielland A, Olsen KM, Christophersen AS. False-positive results with Emit II amphetamine/methamphetamine assay in users of common psychotropic drugs. Clin Chem 1995;41:951–2.

31. Colbert DL. Possible explanation for trimethobenzamide cross-reaction in immunoassays of amphetamine/methamphetamine. Clin Chem 1994;40:948–9.

32. Melanson SE, Baskin L, Magnani B, et al. Interpretation and utility of drug of abuse immunoassays: lessons from laboratory drug testing surveys. Arch Pathol Lab Med 2010;134:735–9.

Drug Testing in the Neonate

Steven W. Cotten, PhD, DABCC

KEYWORDS

- Neonate • Drugs of abuse • Meconium • Pregnancy • Newborn

KEY POINTS

- Drug screening in the newborn population comes with a set of unique analytical, therapeutic, and legal issues that can make testing and result interpretation challenging.
- Assessment of in utero drug exposure to cocaine, amphetamines, opiates, marijuana, and ethanol may allow better intervention and management of withdrawal symptoms for the neonate.
- A range of maternal and neonatal specimens are available, but each comes with a unique set of limitations regarding sensitivity, invasiveness, and window of detection.
- Preanalytical issues such as specimen collection and sample extraction can influence test accuracy, and the particular biological specimen evaluated determines the window of detection achieved.
- Meconium provides the longest window, but the extraction technique greatly impacts sensitivity, and unique drug metabolites in meconium may lead to discrepancies between maternal and neonate results.

INTRODUCTION

A major portion of toxicology testing deals with urine drug screening for the adult population. This group can be divided into two major applications: preemployment urine drug screening and periodic scheduled pain management screening. Pain management clinics usually require patients to sign opiate contracts that allow for regular testing as a means to assess compliance. The presence or absence of drugs and metabolites must match the patient's prescribed medications, and any discrepant compounds found during routine screening are grounds for dismissal from the pain management program. In addition to these two applications, toxicology drug testing plays an important but often overlooked role in newborn drug screening. Testing this population comes with its own set of unique analytical, therapeutic, and legal issues that can make screening and result interpretation challenging.

The author has nothing to disclose.
Department of Pathology and Laboratory Medicine, University of North Carolina at Chapel Hill, 101 Manning Drive, Chapel Hill, NC, 27514, USA
E-mail address: scotten@unch.unc.edu

Clin Lab Med 32 (2012) 449–466
http://dx.doi.org/10.1016/j.cll.2012.06.008
0272-2712/12/$ – see front matter © 2012 Elsevier Inc. All rights reserved.

The rationale for newborn drug screening seeks to establish a picture of prenatal drug exposure during pregnancy. Conventional testing in adults uses both self-reporting and biological specimen testing to provide the necessary information for establishment of compliance or abuse. In the case of newborns, self-reporting is not applicable, and clinicians must rely on information from the mother coupled with biological testing from both the mother and neonate. Additionally, interpretation of drug screening results may be left to physicians, nurses, or social services workers. As the complexity of testing and interpretation increases, it is imperative that the laboratory be proactive in educating the necessary parties involved, particularly those without extensive toxicology training, to ensure proper medical and legal decisions are made with the information provided.

The unique analytical and legal caveats associated with newborn drug testing pose a variety of challenges to laboratorians and clinicians alike when it comes to screening this specific population. Preanalytical issues such as specimen collection and sample extraction can influence test accuracy. Samples can easily be adulterated because of the access of family members to the infant and extensive unsupervised time. Newborns frequently have dilute urine, so false-negatives are likely. Furthermore, sample volume is often low, limiting the ability for comprehensive screening and confirmation testing. Therefore, negative urine results do not definitively rule out drug exposure.

Positive urine results cannot distinguish between intermittent and chronic use by the mother. Often there is low agreement between specimens from the mother and newborn as well as results from screening and confirmation. Instances of discordant results complicates interpretation, particularly in cases with multiple specimens. Several therapeutic issues related to medical management are also unique to this population. The mother may initially delay prenatal care to avoid urine drug testing. Subsequent toxicology results have limited predictive value on genetic changes that have taken place earlier during the pregnancy. Positive drug screening results, however, can allow for proper medical management of withdrawal symptoms for certain drug classes.

Perhaps the most serious issues related to newborn drug testing are the legal implications surrounding decisions made in the case of positive results. Positive urine or meconium drug samples in newborns trigger involvement from social services for assessment of child safety. Twelve states formally consider positive urine drug screen in an infant to be child abuse; therefore, laboratory results can potentially remove newborns from their biological parents and place them in the foster care system. For this reason, the caveats and limitations of drug testing in this population are of utmost importance.

SUBSTANCE ABUSE DURING PREGNANCY

Accurate assessment of substance abuse during pregnancy is challenging for clinicians and other health care workers. Determination of abuse can come from either self-reporting or biological specimen testing. The US Department of Health and Human Services in conjunction with the Substance Abuse and Mental Health Administration periodically conducts surveys on drug use in persons 12 years and older in the general US population. In 2009, data estimated 22.6 million Americans (8.9%) used illicit drugs in the month before the survey.[1] A total of 4.4% of pregnant women ages 15 to 44 admitted to substance abuse in the last month. This rate was lower than nonpregnant women (10.9%) and decreased with the age of respondent. The frequency of substance abuse was 16.2% for women ages 15 to 17, 7.4% for ages 18 to 25, and 1.9% for ages 25 to 55. Alcohol use among pregnant women was estimated at 10.8%, with 3.7% admitting to binge drinking and 1.9% admitting to heavy alcohol use.

When biological specimens from pregnant mothers or newborns are tested for the presence of drugs, the rate of substance abuse detected increases. Using biological specimens, the frequency of illicit drug use in pregnant women has been estimated at 20% using maternal urine, maternal hair, newborn urine, or meconium.[2–4] Tobacco and alcohol use/abuse are also estimated around 19%.

CRITERIA FOR TESTING AND CONSENT

Clinical indication for substance abuse testing is highly variable between regions. Currently there are no federal guidelines defining criteria for the testing of newborns or pregnant women. Therefore, it is up to individual institutions and health care systems to draft explicit guidelines for newborn and maternal drug testing to best identify and manage substance abuse in their specific population. Evidence-based clinical practice guidelines have been developed to provide recommendations for standardized screening approaches.[3,5,6] Typical institutional guidelines for toxicology screening for newborns may resemble the following. (Adapted from the newborn nursery guidelines from the University of North Carolina at Chapel Hill.[7])

Urine or meconium drug testing is clinically indicated by the following:

- Maternal History
  - History of drug abuse.
  - Prenatal care starting after 16 weeks or less than a total of four prenatal visits.
  - History of child abuse, neglect, or court-ordered placement of children outside the home.
  - History of domestic violence.
  - History of hepatitis, human immunodeficiency virus, syphilis, or prostitution.
  - Unexplained placental abruption.

- Infant History
  - Unexplained intrauterine growth restriction.
  - Infants with evidence of drug withdrawal (hypertonia, irritability, or tremulousness).

- Alcohol
  - Acute maternal alcohol intoxication is observed around the time of delivery.

Consent for collection is an additional issue requiring special attention for toxicology testing in this population. Informed consent may be required for both maternal and newborn specimens depending on institutional and state guidelines. Consent for collection of newborn urine or meconium for drug screening is often covered under the general consent for treatment for most health care institutions. Departments of obstetrics and gynecology within the hospital may seek separate verbal consent from the mother and inform the parents prior to testing if drug screening becomes clinically indicated.

LEGAL IMPLICATIONS

Most clinical laboratories do not routinely perform chain of custody for specimens submitted for toxicology analysis. This protocol differs from employment urine drug screening where documentation of chain of custody is necessary for validity of the results. Legal action can be taken only if chain of custody is properly documented. In the case of newborn drug screening, if a specimen is positive for an illicit substance, chain of custody is not required for legal action or involvement by social services. This difference illustrates an important nuance in newborn drug testing in that both

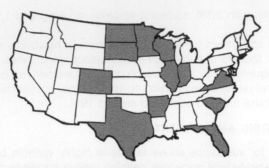

Fig. 1. States that consider a positive newborn urine drug screen child abuse. Arkansas, Colorado, Florida, Illinois, Indiana, Minnesota, North Dakota, South Carolina, South Dakota, Texas, Virginia, Wisconsin, and the District of Columbia incorporate a positive urine drug screen for a newborn in their definition of child abuse.

medical and legal decisions are made using the results generated by the clinical laboratory. It is therefore imperative that all parties involved in the testing process— nurses, medical technologists, physicians, laboratory directors, substance abuse counselors, and social services workers—have a unified protocol for testing and understand the limitations.

A compendium of individual state laws regarding parental drug use and child abuse is available from the Child Welfare Information Gateway.[8] Arkansas, Colorado, Florida, Illinois, Indiana, Minnesota, North Dakota, South Carolina, South Dakota, Texas, Virginia, Wisconsin, and the District of Columbia all consider a positive newborn urine drug screen in their definition of child abuse or neglect (**Fig. 1**). An additional 13 states have specific reporting procedures for newborns that show evidence of exposure to drugs or alcohol. The Child Abuse Prevention and Treatment Act requires states to develop formal policies for informing child protective services in cases where newborn drug exposure is documented and to develop plans for protective care and medical management of withdrawal symptoms.[9]

TYPES OF SPECIMENS

The goal of toxicology drug testing in newborns is to evaluate in utero drug exposure during the course of the pregnancy. A wide range of maternal and neonate biological specimens are available to clinicians. Each specimen comes with its own unique set of limitations regarding sensitivity, invasiveness, and window of detection. Biological matrices from the newborn include meconium, hair, cord blood, and neonate urine. Specimens from the mother include hair, blood, oral fluid, sweat, urine, and breast milk. Matrices that contain drugs and metabolites from both the mother and neonate include the placenta and amniotic fluid. In order to develop a complete understanding of total drug exposure during pregnancy, clinicians must consider the type of specimen being tested, the type of drug expected, and the window of detection (**Fig. 2**). The rate of agreement between mother and infant can often be low because of these complicating factors.

SPECIMENS FROM THE NEONATE

The three types of commonly used specimens from the newborn include neonate urine, neonate hair, and meconium. Neonate urine is the most frequently used

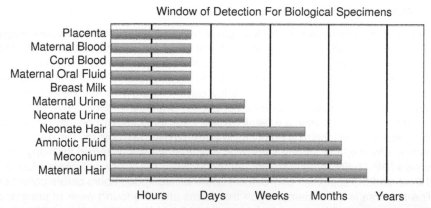

Fig. 2. Window of detection for biological specimens: The window of detection varies depending on the sample chosen for drugs of abuse screening. (*From* Lozano J, García-Algar O, Vall O, et al. Biological matrices for the evaluation of in utero exposure to drugs of abuse. Ther Drug Monit 2007;29:711–34, **Figure 2**; with permission.)

specimen to assess in utero drug exposure. Despite its popularity, urine samples provide the shortest window of detection, only capturing drug use several days before delivery.[10] Newborns also tend to have dilute urine, so false-negatives are likely.

Neonate hair forms during the last trimester, and therefore can capture drug exposure for the last 3 to 4 months during pregnancy.[11] The parent compounds of drugs typically accumulate in hair rather than the more polar metabolites found in blood, urine, and meconium through either passive diffusion from arterial blood capillaries of the hair follicle or excretion on the surface of the head. Typically 20 to 50 mg of hair are needed for adequate testing, but because quantities may be limited in newborns and the procedure is considered partially invasive, adoption of hair testing has not gained routine usage.[12]

Meconium refers to the first fecal matter passed during the first days of life; it is characterized by a dark green/black color. Formation of meconium begins around the 12th week of gestation and continues to accumulate until birth.[13] Drugs of abuse are deposited in meconium through absorbance across the placenta, metabolism by the fetal liver, and swallowing of amniotic fluid.[14,15] The length of accumulation imparts the largest window of detection for drugs of abuse for any neonate specimen, theoretically capturing the entire profile of exposure over the last two trimesters.

Collection of meconium is considered noninvasive, with 99% of full-term infants passing their entire meconium after 48 hours. Drug-exposed neonates show a slower evacuation of meconium, with the median first stool passing at day 3 and 90% by day 12.[16] For analysis, a minimum of 0.5 grams is collected and stored at $-20°C$ to $-80°C$ prior to organic solvent extraction and measurement. The choice of solvent depends on the compound measured and the subsequent method used for analysis. Methanol is the most common extraction solvent for cocaine, opiates, cannabinoids, and amphetamines when liquid chromatography–mass spectrometry (LCMS) is used, with extraction efficiencies between 40% and 80% depending on the individual metabolite assayed. Extraction under acidic conditions may increase recovery through hydrolysis of glucuronide metabolites at a low pH. *The extraction procedure for recovery of drug metabolites from meconium samples has a much greater effect on assay sensitivity than the screening or confirmation procedure itself.*

SPECIMENS FROM THE MOTHER

Biological specimens available for toxicology testing from the mother include maternal hair, urine, blood, amniotic fluid, placenta, cord blood, and oral fluid. Of these specimens, maternal hair and urine are used most frequently during pregnancy and immediately after delivery to assess drug use by the mother. Maternal blood only captures acute consumption occurring a few days or hours prior to collection and has found limited value in testing for drugs of abuse. Oral fluid is noninvasive compared with blood, and drugs that are weak bases such as cocaine, opiates, benzodiazepines, and nicotine tend to accumulate in oral fluid relative to serum. The distribution, detection window, and analyte stability in oral fluid are still unknown for many drugs of abuse.[17,18] Generally only parent compounds are the major component found in oral fluid, and the specimen only detects acute consumption hours before collection.

The placenta is the maternal organ that forms after the fourth week of pregnancy and acts as the interface between maternal and fetal blood, allowing for exchange of nutrients and waste during development. Metabolism and degradation of xenobiotics by the placenta can also occur and impact drug transfer to fetus. Biomarkers of ethanol use by the mother, namely fatty acid ethyl esters (FAEEs), are not transferred to the fetus but are instead absorbed and degraded by the placenta.[19] Therefore, any FAEEs detected in the neonate are a result of direct exposure to ethanol and metabolism by the fetus in utero. Despite its important role in drug metabolism and exposure during pregnancy, placenta testing remains an esoteric specimen used in toxicology testing.

Amniotic fluid accumulates throughout pregnancy, having a volume of approximately 30 mL at week 10 and up to 1000 mL by week 37.[20] The highly aqueous nature of the specimen selectively enriches for water-soluble drugs. Collection of amniotic fluid, however, can be dangerous for the fetus, and its use for drug testing is not routine. Despite this obstacle, several studies have used amniotic fluid to confirm cocaine exposure, but its popularity as a biological fluid for prenatal drug use remains low.[21-24]

The two most popular biological specimens from the mother for assessing prenatal drug exposure are maternal hair and urine. Maternal hair captures chronic drug use over the longest period of time. Collection is noninvasive and provides a direct estimate of maternal drug exposure throughout the entire pregnancy or before. Drug deposition in the hair may, however, be affected by hair care products or cosmetic hair treatments that damage the follicle or hair proteins.[25] Maternal hair analysis provides only an indirect estimation of drug exposure for the fetus. Several studies have attempted to correlate cocaine concentrations between maternal and neonate hair with unpredictable results.[26] Maternal urine in conjunction with neonate urine is probably the most popular specimen to assess drug exposure several days before delivery. Despite its short window of detection, collection is easy, extraction is efficient, and sensitivities in the ng/mL can be achieved for most drugs tested using LC or gas chromatography–mass spectrometry (GCMS).

AGREEMENT BETWEEN MATERNAL AND NEONATE SPECIMENS

Immunoassay screening and mass spectrometry (MS) confirmation results for both maternal and neonate specimens, along with maternal self-reporting, may show varying degrees of agreement. Several factors contribute to these discrepancies. Maternal self-reporting is estimated to capture only 4% of illicit drug users from a general population. Urine specimens from both the mother and neonate have a narrow window of detection for most drugs and are greatly affected by hydration status. In the case of meconium, extraction efficiency and completeness of collection may negatively select for drug detection. Furthermore, if GCMS is used for confirmation, extraction, derivatization, and volatilization will not be equal for different drug classes and their respectively glucuronidated metabolites. Comparing results from different matrices (maternal urine vs neonate meconium) often shows the presence of certain drugs in one specimen that are absent in another.

SPECIMEN COLLECTION AS A SOURCE OF PREANALYTICAL VARIABILITY

In addition to distinctive specimens used in newborn testing, collection methods for urine and meconium are unique. These newborn-specific factors may contribute to preanalytical variability that can affect assay results. The physical collection of urine specimens from newborns is often overlooked as a source of preanalytical variability. A recent study illustrated a wide range of collection procedures in place for neonate urine collection at one institution.[27] Nursing staff at this institution used specially designed urine bags, diapers turned inside-out, cotton balls, or gauze followed by syringe extraction from the textile matrix to collect the urine specimen prior to sending the sample to the laboratory. In some instances the infant was given a bath prior to application of the collection device, whereas other times baby wipes were used. As a result a variety of textiles including diapers, baby wipes, gauze, and lotions could potentially come in contact with the sample prior to analysis.

It is therefore important to validate the collection procedure to identify interferences that may generate false-positives or false-negatives. A false-positive interference from baby wash soaps has recently been reported for several tetrahydrocannabinol (THC) immunoassays for cannabinoids.[27] The interferent was identified after an increase in positive specimens was observed specifically from the institution's newborn nursery. This result can be problematic because confirmatory testing is not mandated in the clinical setting. The interferent was found to be analyte- and manufacturer-dependent. A variety of other household chemicals, namely liquid soap and Visine, have previously been reported as positive interferents in drugs of abuse assays in the context of adulterants for preemployment screening but not in the newborn population.[28,29]

METHODS FOR SCREENING AND CONFIRMATION

Conventional urine drug toxicology consists first of a broad screening method that detects a class of related compounds followed by confirmation of positive results with a second method that detects a defined list of compounds within that class. Regardless of the matrix, urine drug screening almost exclusively uses immunoassay-based platforms that target cocaine, amphetamines, cannabinoids, opiates, or phencyclidine. Clinical laboratories confirm presumptive positive results using MS coupled with LC or GC that imparts increased sensitivity and specificity for quantitating a specific set of compounds. Given the medical and legal decisions that potentially impact patient care and the unique specimens associated with neonate drug screening, it is recommended that all toxicology screening results for drugs of abuse be confirmed.

SPECIFIC DRUGS OF ABUSE
Cocaine

Illicit drug use including cocaine among pregnant women is estimated at 4% based on national studies.[1] After ingestion via smoking or insufflation, cocaine enters the blood where it can be metabolized by the liver or rapidly cross the placenta via

Cocaine Metabolism

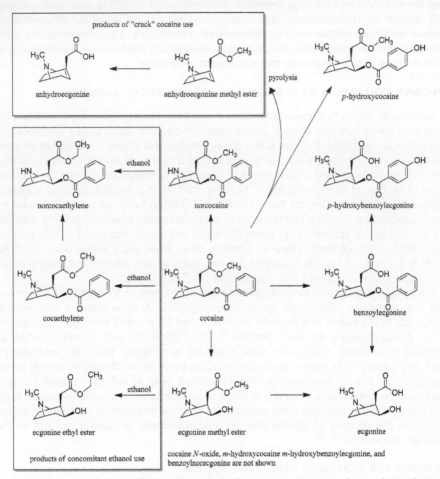

Fig. 3. Cocaine metabolism: The cocaine metabolites present in a sample are dependent on concomitant ethanol use, route of administration, and the biological specimen evaluated.

passive diffusion. Several important metabolic pathways for cocaine are recognized (**Fig. 3**). The various metabolites have a diverse range of polarities and therefore are not uniformly enriched in meconium.[30,31] Cocaine, norcocaine, *p*-hydroxycocaine, benzoylecgonine, ecgonine methyl ester, ecgonine, anhydroecgonine methyl ester, cocaethylene, and norcocaethylene are the major metabolites frequently found in meconium. Interestingly, ecgonine has been shown to occur at the highest frequency and median level for cocaine-exposure infants using solid phase extraction of the meconium.[30] Evaluation of cocaine metabolism for either meta or para hydroxylation showed para hydroxylation to occur at a higher frequency in samples. Median values for meta hydroxylation (*m*-hydroxycocaine or *m*-hydroxybenzoylecgonine), however, exceeded median values for their corresponding para metabolites when present.[30]

Concomitant use of ethanol and cocaine generates the ethyl derivatives norcocaethylene, cocaethylene, and ecgonine ethyl ester via transesterification with ethyl alcohol instead of water. Two specific metabolites can be used to differentiate insufflated cocaine from smoked (crack) cocaine. The pyrolytic products anhydroecgonine methyl ester and anhydroecgonine are both generated directly from the loss of benzoic acid by cocaine during volatilization. The frequency of detection for both ethanol- and crack cocaine–associated metabolites is greater than 95% in the meconium of infants whose mother's urinalysis was positive for benzoylecgonine.[30]

Conventional methods for both immunoassay and MS confirmation target benzoylecgonine, the major ionic metabolite of cocaine found in urine. Current immunoassays effectively recognize both benzoylecgonine and m-hydroxybenzoylecgonine but show little reactivity toward cocaine, ecgonine methyl ester, ecgonine, or cocaethylene.[32] This result may account for some discrepant values between neonate and mother dyads in regard to positive or negative result agreement.

Methanol extraction of meconium is frequently used for isolation of cocaine metabolites. This extraction can be coupled with solid phase extraction to further enrich additional compounds other than benzoylecgonine through reconstitution in acidic buffer followed by additional washing and elution in methylene chloride/2-propanol-ammonium hydroxide (78/20/2).[30] This inclusive extraction procedure has reported recoveries of 15 unique cocaine metabolites between 38.9% and 59.1%.

Immunoassay-based screening methods including radioimmunoassay, enzyme-multiplied immunoassay technique (EMIT), enzyme-linked immunosorbent assay, and fluorescence polarization have all been used for cocaine determination with neonate urine and meconium.[12] GC and LCMS methodologies have been adopted for confirmation testing of meconium samples allowing for quantitation of comprehensive panels of cocaine metabolites. LCMS methods achieve greater sensitivity than GCMS because of elimination of the derivatization and volatilization steps required by gas chromatography.

Effects of in utero cocaine exposure

A large epidemiologic study of 11,811 mother-infant pairs compared meconium and maternal self-reporting to assess drug exposure.[33] Of the analyzed samples, 9.5% were positive for cocaine or its metabolites using EMIT immunoassay followed by GCMS. At birth, neonate exposure to cocaine was significantly associated with low birth weight and altered length and head circumference from normal ranges.[34] Additionally, prenatal cocaine exposure has been linked to delayed language development, decreased total language performance, behavior problems in school, and increased risk of obesity through early adolescence.[35,36]

Cannabinoids

Cannabinoids are a class of compounds produced by Cannabis sativa and Cannabis indica with Δ^9-THC being the most prevalent and the major psychoactive component. Assessment of prenatal cannabis exposure relies on maternal self-reporting, maternal urine, neonate urine, and meconium. Metabolism of THC generates 11-nor-Δ9-tetrahydrocannabinol-9-carboxylic acid (THC-COOH) through the active intermediate 11-hydroxy-Δ9-tetrahydrocannabinol (11-OH-THC). The majority of immunoassays target THC-COOH because it is the major constituent in cannabinoid-positive urine samples.[37] Meconium does, however, have a greater likelihood of detecting sporadic cannabis use during pregnancy; it is often preferred over newborn urine (**Fig. 4**).

Differences in cannabinoid metabolite content exist between urine and meconium in the neonate that can lead to high rates of false-negatives. Studies evaluating meconium samples that screen positive by EMIT assay but confirm negative for THC-COOH revealed a 40% false-positive rate.[38] Further analysis of meconium

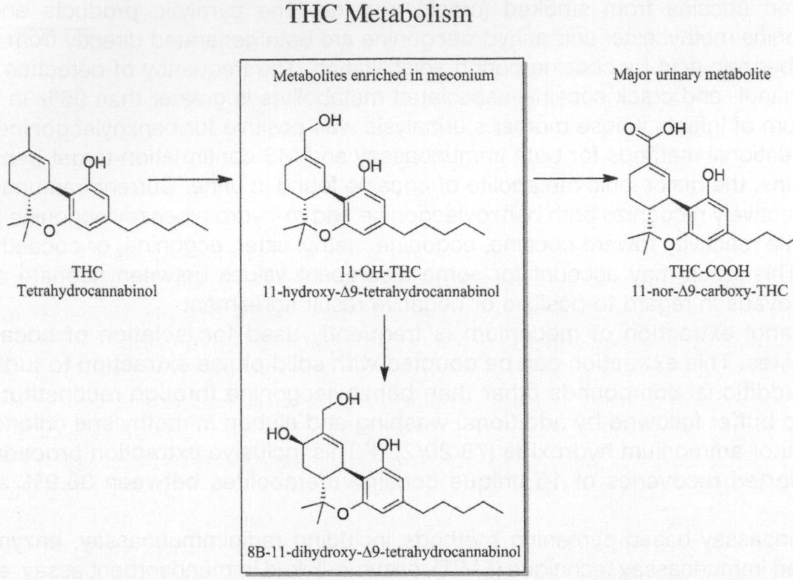

THC Metabolism

Fig. 4. THC metabolism: In addition to the major urinary metabolite THC-COOH, meconium may selectively accumulate 11-OH-THC and 8β-11-dihydroxy-Δ9-tetrahydrocannabinol as a result of maternal THC use during pregnancy.

samples that screened negative for THC-COOH detected 11-OH-THC and 8β-11-dihydroxy-Δ9-tetrahydrocannabinol (8β-di-OH-THC) instead.[38,39] These data suggest that meconium may selectively enrich distinct cannabinoid metabolites from urine, and that confirmation rates can be increased by incorporation of these additional compounds (see Fig. 4).

A dose-response relationship between maternal drug use and neonate meconium cannabinoid concentration has not been established, making estimation of maternal episodic use difficult. Serial collection of meconium samples over the first several days has demonstrated a 60% likelihood of a subsequent positive result if the first collected sample is positive.[14] This issue highlights the heterogeneous nature of meconium collection and how the dynamics of gastrointestinal motility can affect test results.

Sample preparation for cannabinoid extraction from meconium can be achieved using normal saline, methanol, acetic acid/diphenylamine, or hexane/ethyl acetate.[40–43] Methanol extraction and subsequent analysis of THC-COOH can yield recoveries between 50% and 72%.[39] THC and its metabolites are glucuronidated in both urine and meconium; therefore, enzymatic, acid or base hydrolysis improves sensitivities for GC or LCMS.

Interferences in THC-COOH immunoassay assays have been reported on a variety of manufacturer platforms.[27,29,44] Newborn-specific factors related to sample collection (urine) may also impart preanalytical variation for THC immunoassay results.[27] To complicate immunoassay interpretation there are three prescription drugs that contain cannabinoid-based molecules. Medicinal marijuana is available by prescription in one out of three states in the United States, the pain management drug Marinol (THC) is given to specific pain populations, and the new neurologic agent (Sativex, THC/cannabidiol) is used for the treatment of multiple sclerosis. Although there are no recommendations for use of the medications during pregnancy, drug screening results should be critically evaluated if the mother has a medical history involving any of these prescription drugs.

Effects of in utero cannabinoid exposure

Numerous studies have sought to measure quantitatively the effects of maternal cannabis use on neonate development. Several studies have reported negative physical effects on birth weight, length, and gestational age.[45,46] Below-normal performance on intelligence tests, increased frequency of depression, and greater likelihood to use cannabis in adolescence have also been associated with prenatal exposure.[47-49] Yet other studies find no adverse effects at birth or demonstrable long-term differences between exposed and nonexposed neonates.[50-52] Such discrepant findings have been suggested to arise from inability to properly stratify exposed from nonexposed infants.[53] Despite a lack of conclusive evidence for or against harmful effects of prenatal THC exposure, substance abuse often correlates with other environmental and social factors that can negatively affect development.

Opiates

The frequency and amount of opiate consumption has increased dramatically in the past decade. Drug screening has become increasingly complex as the need to discriminate between over-the-counter, prescription, and illicit opiates grows in the clinical setting. The rapid emergence of pain management clinics now requires specific quantitation of multiple prescription opiates to assess patient compliance. In the setting of pregnancy, opiate testing is important for both maternal and neonate health, particularly for opiate-dependent mothers and the proper management of neonate abstinence syndrome at birth.

The type of opiate molecule in question will determine its immunoassay reactivity, transport across the placenta, and tissue distribution in the neonate. Morphine-based opiates such as morphine, codeine, oxycodone, hydrocodone, buprenorphine, and heroin are lipophilic and will be transferred readily across the placenta to the fetus. Their corresponding glucuronidated metabolites are more hydrophilic and will cross the placenta via diffusion-limited transfer.[54] The rate of diffusion is gated by the size of the molecule as well as the permeability of the placenta, which changes with gestational age. Based on animal studies, synthetic opiates such as fentanyl, methadone, tramadol, and loperamide may exhibit greater transfer across the placenta than morphine-based drugs and subsequent increased fetal exposure.[55]

Opiate metabolism generates glucuronidated compounds that are found in both urine and meconium. Neonate urine samples provide a narrow window of detection of maternal drug use in the past 3 to 7 days. For heroin, the generation of 6-monoacetylmorphine is only detectable hours after use before the intermediate is converted entirely to morphine. The major cyclic metabolite of methadone, 2-ethylidene-1,5-dimethyl-3,3-diphenyl-pyrrolidine (EDDP), has been detected in meconium using fluorescence polarization and high-performance LC with diode array detection.[56] A correlation was seen with the maternal methadone dose and the amount of meconium methadone measured but not with the methadone metabolite EDDP.

Immunoassay reactivity toward opiates varies depending on manufacturer, platform, and target compound. Semisynthetic morphine–based opiates such as oxycodone and buprenorphine may show partial reactivity, whereas nonmorphine–based opiates such as methadone and fentanyl may not react at all. Methanolic extraction of meconium is frequently used for isolation of opiates from the specimen prior to analysis. Extensive coverage of the methodologies and detection limits for a variety of opiate assays in the setting of neonate drug testing has been reviewed elsewhere.[12]

Neonate abstinence syndrome

Methadone is currently the only approved medication for use during pregnancy by opioid-dependent women.[57] Maintenance therapy for pregnant women is thought to reduce illicit drug–seeking behavior, minimize withdrawal-induced stress on the fetus, and improve prenatal care. Maternal methadone use exposes the neonate to opiates during gestation, which can present central and autonomic nervous system dysfunction at birth, frequently called neonate abstinence syndrome (NAS). Assessment depends on observed behaviors such as excessive crying, poor sleep, tremors, increased muscle tone, generalized seizure, hyperthermia, tachypnea, poor feeding, failure to thrive, and irritability. Pharmacologic management depends on degree of severity, with 52% of NAS patients requiring only opiates for treatment.[58] Second line therapies include phenobarbital and opiates in 32% of cases. Buprenorphine has recently been reported as a safe and effective treatment for NAS, along with clonidine.[59,60]

Amphetamines

Amphetamine drug testing in the neonate is similar to opiate testing in that it must discriminate between over-the-counter, prescription, and illicit compounds within the same class. Immunoassay screening serves only to capture the maximum number of true-positives for reflex confirmation testing while minimizing false-positives. Specificity of reagents and platforms varies for amphetamine drugs of abuse detection. It is therefore up to laboratories to educate health care professionals in proper test utility and institution-specific limitations.

Methamphetamine abuse has increased sharply in specific regions of the country over the last 10 years, with 11,239 clandestine laboratories discovered in 2010.[61] Tennessee, Kentucky, and Illinois account for 30% of the total manufacturing of methamphetamine in the United States. Approximately 17% to 44% of laboratories have children living in the same building. In the last several years, a shift in the synthetic route used for the manufacturing of methamphetamine has occurred that allows for small-scale mobile manufacture in 2 L bottles. The method known as "shake and bake" has increased the number of amateur producers and subsequently burn victims admitted to hospitals.

Maternal use of methamphetamine increased from 8% in 1994 to 24% in 2006 for pregnant women positive for an illicit substance.[62] Methamphetamine crosses the placenta within 30 seconds of injection in animal studies and exhibits slower elimination in the fetus resulting in longer exposure. Heavy prenatal use of methamphetamine is associated with high concentrations (200–1000 ng/g) in meconium. Amphetamines, including methamphetamine, MDMA (methylenedioxymethamphetamine), and MDA (methylenedioxyamphetamine) can be deaminated or hydroxylated in the liver to inactive metabolites. Unlike other drug classes, a significant portion (30%–40%) is excreted unchanged in the urine, making detection of the parent compound acceptable for assessing exposure. Detection in neonate urine captures exposure several days before birth. False-positive results from labetalol, a drug used to treat hypertension during pregnancy, have been reported, highlighting the need for confirmation of positive immunoassay screening results from maternal urine.[63]

Methanolic extraction often coupled with solid phase purification is used for extraction of amphetamines from meconium.[42] Confirmation by GC and LCMS offers sensitivities in the ng range per gram of meconium. Extraction efficiencies between

Fatty Acid Ethyl Ester Biosynthesis

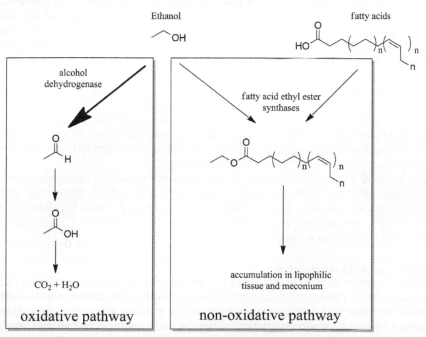

Fig. 5. Fatty acid ethyl ester biosynthesis: FAEEs are generated in the nonoxidative breakdown of ethanol. Reaction of ethanol with endogenous fatty acids generating FAEEs and their accumulation in meconium may be a good indicator of maternal ethanol use during pregnancy.

40% and 87% have been reported across a wide range of concentrations. Additionally, specific byproducts of methamphetamine production have been used in the forensic setting to determine which route was used for synthesis.[61,64]

Side effects of prenatal methamphetamine and amphetamine exposure include decreased gestational age, birth weight, length, and occipitofrontal circumference.[62] Additionally, infants are more likely to be admitted to neonate intensive care units after birth. Beyond initial clinical effects, decreases in mother-infant bonding, decreases in breast-feeding, higher adoption rates, neglect, and court-ordered placement outside the home are associated with mothers who use methamphetamine.[65]

Ethanol

Assessment of ethanol abuse during pregnancy is challenging because of rapid metabolism and elimination by the body.[66] The pseudo-zero order kinetics and rapid distribution throughout tissues make detection in the blood and urine difficult. Diagnostic tests to assay neonate exposure to alcohol are currently evaluating the emerging biomarkers of FAEEs, which are produced through nonoxidative breakdown of ethanol (**Fig. 5**).[67] Normal reaction of fatty acids with glycerol in the body produces monoglycerides, diglycerides, and triglycerides that act as secondary messengers and cellular components. In the presence of ethanol, fatty acids form FAEEs through a condensation reaction. Once formed, FAEEs are deposited in fatty tissues and meconium, thereby serving as markers for long-term alcohol exposure during pregnancy.

Studies evaluating transfer of FAEEs across the placenta demonstrate that FAEEs generated by maternal metabolism are broken down and degraded in the placenta.[19] Accumulation of FAEEs in meconium, therefore, represents ethanol that has been transferred across the placenta and metabolized by the fetus in utero. The major FAEEs currently under evaluation include ethyl laurate, ethyl myristate, ethyl palmitate, ethyl palmitoleate, ethyl stearate, ethyl oleate, ethyl linoleate, ethyl alpha-linoleate, ethyl arachidonate, and ethyl heptadecanoate.[68]

Correlation between maternal alcohol consumption and FAEEs levels in meconium show a positive relationship, but the specific analytes and cutoff levels defining exposure remain unclear. Total FAEEs levels are suggested to provide better predictive power for maternal alcohol abuse rather than select individual metabolites. Furthermore, the cutoff levels for positive prenatal alcohol exposure vary by study, with reported cutoffs ranging from 50 to 600 ng/g.[66]

Extraction of FAEEs from meconium has been achieved with hexane/acetone or solid phase extraction with recoveries ranging from 20% to 93% depending on the specific metabolite tested. Testing methods have used GC–flame ion detector, full scan GC-MS, selected ion monitoring GC-MS, and GC-MS/MS for screening and confirmation of various analytes.

Fetal alcohol spectrum disorder

Prenatal exposure to alcohol can result in a broad array of detrimental effects to the developing fetus. Fetal alcohol spectrum disorder (FASD) is the umbrella term used to classify neonates that exhibit one or more of the features associated with ethanol exposure including growth retardation, abnormal facial features, and central nervous system impairment.[69] Height and weight below the 10th percentile, short palpebral fissures, thin vermillion border, smooth philtrum, and impaired cognitive function are all used as criteria for diagnosis of FASD. It is estimated that the occurrence of FASD is between 0.2 and 2 cases per 1000 births in the United States.[69] Secondary effects that may present later in life include legal trouble, mental health issues, behavioral problems, and low social adaptability. The cost of FASD has been estimated at $3.6 billion annually, illustrating its severity as a major public health issue.

MANAGEMENT OF WITHDRAWAL FROM DRUGS OF ABUSE

Guidelines for medical management for chronic prenatal exposure to opiates, benzodiazepine, and alcohol have been proposed by the SOGC[5] (**Table 1**). Neonates showing abstinence syndrome from opiates can benefit from symptomatic therapy, including Gravol for nausea and vomiting and acetaminophen/nonsteroidal antiinflammatory drugs for myalgias. Methadone and buprenorphine can be initiated to step-down opiate exposure over time. If methadone is unavailable, morphine 5 to 10 mg by mouth every 4 to 6 hours as needed can be substituted. For chronic benzodiazepine exposure, two-thirds to three-fourths of the equivalent adult dose (mg/kg) can be administered, tapering 10% of the dose per day. Chronic alcohol exposure withdrawal can benefit from thiamine, folic acid, diazepam, or lorazepam depending on severity, with close monitoring of electrolytes.

FUTURE PERSPECTIVES

The neonate population holds unique challenges in relation to assessment of drug exposure. The specimens available show distinct differences from adult samples regarding windows of detection and analyte deposition. Accurate results are imperative given the legal and medical management issues related to newborn care.

Table 1
Management of withdrawal symptoms

Substance	Recommended Management
Alcohol	Thiamine 100 mg po od × 3 d, folic acid 5 mg po od. Diazepam 20 mg po q 1–2 h until minimal symptoms. Lorazepam 2–4 mg sl/po q 2–4 h prn during labor. Monitor hydration status.
Benzodiazepines	Start at two-thirds to three-fourths of diazepam equivalent dose. Taper by 10% per day.
Opiates	Offer symptomatic therapy including Gravol for nausea and vomiting, acetaminophen/NSAIDs for myalgias. Consider methadone or buprenorphine initiation. Can use morphine 5–10 mg po q 4–6 h prn if methadone is not available.

Abbreviations: NSAIDs, nonsteroidal antiinflammatory drugs; od, once daily; po, by mouth; prn, as needed; q, every; sl, sublingual.
Data from Wong S, Ordean A, Kahan M. SOGC clinical practice guidelines: substance use in pregnancy: no. 256. Int J Gynaecol Obstet 2011;114:190–202.

Current research in the area of FAEEs may provide better tools to evaluate prenatal alcohol exposure in the future. Several additional facets of neonate drug testing deserve more research to understand exposure rates more clearly and detrimental effects of drugs during development. To date, little information exists regarding the frequency and level of the cocaine adulterant levamisole in meconium. Current estimates for levamisole prevalence in the adult population are approaching 100% for patients who screen positive for benzoylecgonine. Additionally, the synthetic cannabinoids and novel ketone amphetamines currently emerging in adult populations have not been evaluated in the neonate population.

REFERENCES

1. US Department of Health and Human Services. Results from the 2010 National Survey on Drug Use and Health: summary of national findings. Substance Abuse and Mental Health Services Administration report No. SMA 11-4658. 2011. Available at: http://oas.samhsa.gov/NSDUH/2k10NSDUH/2k10Results.htm. Accessed April 10, 2012.
2. Havens JR, Simmons LA, Shannon LM, et al. Factors associated with substance use during pregnancy: results from a national sample. Drug Alcohol Depend 2009;99:89–95.
3. Yonkers KA, Gotman N, Kershaw T, et al. Screening for prenatal substance use: development of the Substance Use Risk Profile-Pregnancy scale. Obstet Gynecol 2010;116:827–33.
4. Substance abuse in pregnancy. The global library of women's medicine. Published 2009. Available at: http://www.glowm.com/?p=glowm.cml/section_view&articleid=115. Accessed April 10, 2012.
5. Wong S, Ordean A, Kahan M. SOGC clinical practice guidelines: substance use in pregnancy: no. 256. Int J Gynaecol Obstet 2011;114:190–202.
6. Murphy-Oikonen J, Montelpare WJ, Southon S, et al. Identifying infants at risk for neonatal abstinence syndrome: a retrospective cohort comparison study of 3 screening approaches. J Perinat Neonatal Nurs 2010;24:366–72.

7. University of North Carolina Department of Labor and Delivery. Clinical guidelines for urine toxicology screening. Chapel Hill (NC): University of North Carolina Department of Labor and Delivery; 2011.
8. Child Welfare Information Gateway. Parental drug use as child abuse. Published 2009. Available at: http://www.childwelfare.gov/systemwide/laws_policies/statutes/drugexposed.cfm. Accessed April 10, 2012.
9. US Department of Health and Human Services. Child Abuse Prevention and Treatment Act. Available at: http://www.acf.hhs.gov/programs/cb/laws_policies/cblaws/capta/. Accessed April 10, 2012.
10. Farst KJ, Valentine JL, Hall RW. Drug testing for newborn exposure to illicit substances in pregnancy: pitfalls and pearls. Int J Pediatr 2011;2011:951616.
11. Gallardo E, Queiroz JA. The role of alternative specimens in toxicological analysis. Biomed Chromatogr 2008;22:795–821.
12. Lozano J, García-Algar O, Vall O, et al. Biological matrices for the evaluation of in utero exposure to drugs of abuse. Ther Drug Monit 2007;29:711–34.
13. Browne SP, Tebbett IR, Moore CM, et al. Analysis of meconium for cocaine in neonates. J Chromatogr 1992;575:158–61.
14. Ostrea EM Jr, Romero A, Knapp DK, et al. Postmortem drug analysis of meconium in early-gestation human fetuses exposed to cocaine: clinical implications. J Pediatr 1994;124:477–9.
15. Kwong TC, Ryan RM. Detection of intrauterine illicit drug exposure by newborn drug testing. National Academy of Clinical Biochemistry. Clin Chem 1997;43:235–42.
16. Verma A, Dhanireddy R. Time of first stool in extremely low birth weight (< or = 1000 grams) infants. J Pediatr 1993;122:626–9.
17. Cone EJ, Clarke J, Tsanaclis L. Prevalence and disposition of drugs of abuse and opioid treatment drugs in oral fluid. J Anal Toxicol 2007;31:424–33.
18. Bosker WM, Huestis MA. Oral fluid testing for drugs of abuse. Clin Chem 2009;55:1910–31.
19. Chan D, Knie B, Boskovic R, et al. Placental handling of fatty acid ethyl esters: perfusion and subcellular studies. J Pharmacol Exp Ther 2004;310:75–82.
20. Sadler T. Langman's Medical Embryology. 12th edition. Philadelphia: Lippincott Williams & Wilkins; 2011. p. 106.
21. Winecker RE, Goldberger BA, Tebbett I, et al. Detection of cocaine and its metabolites in amniotic fluid and umbilical cord tissue. J Anal Toxicol 1997;21:97–104.
22. Ripple MG, Goldberger BA, Caplan YH, et al. Detection of cocaine and its metabolites in human amniotic fluid. J Anal Toxicol 1992;16:328–31.
23. Jain L, Meyer W, Moore C, et al. Detection of fetal cocaine exposure by analysis of amniotic fluid. Obstet Gynecol 1993;81:787–90.
24. Casanova OQ, Lombardero N, Behnke M, et al. Detection of cocaine exposure in the neonate. Analyses of urine, meconium, and amniotic fluid from mothers and infants exposed to cocaine. Arch Pathol Lab Med 1994;118:988–93.
25. Marques PR, Tippetts AS, Branch DG. Cocaine in the hair of mother-infant pairs: quantitative analysis and correlations with urine measures and self-report. Am J Drug Alcohol Abuse 1993;19:159–75.
26. Potter S, Klein J, Valiante G, et al. Maternal cocaine use without evidence of fetal exposure. J Pediatr 1994;125:652–4.
27. Cotten SW, Duncan DL, Burch EA, et al. Unexpected interference of baby wash products with a cannabinoid (THC) immunoassay. Clin Biochem 2012;45(9):605–9.
28. Uebel RA, Wium CA. Toxicological screening for drugs of abuse in samples adulterated with household chemicals. S Afr Med J 2002;92:547–9.

29. Mikkelsen SL, Ash KO. Adulterants causing false negatives in illicit drug testing. Clin Chem 1988;34:2333–6.

30. Xia Y, Wang P, Bartlett MG, et al. An LC-MS-MS method for the comprehensive analysis of cocaine and cocaine metabolites in meconium. Anal Chem 2000;72: 764–71.

31. Murphey LJ, Olsen GD, Konkol RJ. Quantitation of benzoylnorecgonine and other cocaine metabolites in meconium by high-performance liquid chromatography. J Chromatogr 1993;613:330–5.

32. Vitros Chemistry. Cocaine metabolite immunoassay reagent. Rochester (NY): Ortho Clinical Diagnostics; 2010.

33. Bada HS, Das A, Bauer CR, et al. Gestational cocaine exposure and intrauterine growth: maternal lifestyle study. Obstet Gynecol 2002;100:916–24.

34. Bauer CR, Shankaran S, Bada HS, et al. The Maternal Lifestyle Study: drug exposure during pregnancy and short-term maternal outcomes. Am J Obstet Gynecol 2002; 186:487–95.

35. Bandstra ES, Morrow CE, Accornero VH, et al. Estimated effects of in utero cocaine exposure on language development through early adolescence. Neurotoxicol Teratol 2011;33:25–35.

36. Bada HS, Bann CM, Bauer CR, et al. Preadolescent behavior problems after prenatal cocaine exposure: relationship between teacher and caretaker ratings (Maternal Lifestyle Study). Neurotoxicol Teratol 2011;33:78–87.

37. Vitros Chemistry. THC immunoassay reagent. Rochester (NY): Ortho Clinical Diagnostics; 2010.

38. ElSohly MA, Feng S. Delta 9-THC metabolites in meconium: identification of 11-OH-delta 9-THC, 8 beta,11-diOH-delta 9-THC, and 11-nor-delta 9-THC-9-COOH as major metabolites of delta 9-THC. J Anal Toxicol 1998;22:329–35.

39. Feng S, ElSohly MA, Salamone S, et al. Simultaneous analysis of delta9-THC and its major metabolites in urine, plasma, and meconium by GC-MS using an immunoaffinity extraction procedure. J Anal Toxicol 2000;24:395–402.

40. Maynard EC, Amoruso LP, Oh W. Meconium for drug testing. Am J Dis Child 1991;145:650–2.

41. Bar-Oz B, Klein J, Karaskov T, et al. Comparison of meconium and neonatal hair analysis for detection of gestational exposure to drugs of abuse. Arch Dis Child Fetal Neonatal Ed 2003;88:F98–100.

42. ElSohly MA, Stanford DF, Murphy TP, et al. Immunoassay and GC-MS procedures for the analysis of drugs of abuse in meconium. J Anal Toxicol 1999;23:436–45.

43. Moore C, Lewis D, Becker J, et al. The determination of 11-nor-delta 9-tetrahydro-cannabinol-9-carboxylic acid (THCCOOH) in meconium. J Anal Toxicol 1996;20: 50–1.

44. Warner A. Interference of common household chemicals in immunoassay methods for drugs of abuse. Clin Chem 1989;35:648–51.

45. Hatch EE, Bracken MB. Effect of marijuana use in pregnancy on fetal growth. Am J Epidemiol 1986;124:986–93.

46. El Marroun H, Tiemeier H, Steegers EA, et al. Intrauterine cannabis exposure affects fetal growth trajectories: the Generation R Study. J Am Acad Child Adolesc Psychiatry 2009;48:1173–81.

47. Goldschmidt L, Richardson GA, Willford J, et al. Prenatal marijuana exposure and intelligence test performance at age 6. J Am Acad Child Adolesc Psychiatry 2008;47: 254–63.

48. Gray KA, Day NL, Leech S, et al. Prenatal marijuana exposure: effect on child depressive symptoms at ten years of age. Neurotoxicol Teratol 2005;27:439–48.

49. Day NL, Goldschmidt L, Thomas CA. Prenatal marijuana exposure contributes to the prediction of marijuana use at age 14. Addiction 2006;101:1313–22.
50. Dreher MC, Nugent K, Hudgins R. Prenatal marijuana exposure and neonatal outcomes in Jamaica: an ethnographic study. Pediatrics 1994;93:254–60.
51. Lester BM, Dreher M. Effects of marijuana use during pregnancy on newborn cry. Child Dev 1989;60:765–71.
52. van Gelder MM, Reefhuis J, Caton AR, et al. Characteristics of pregnant illicit drug users and associations between cannabis use and perinatal outcome in a population-based study. Drug Alcohol Depend 2010;109:243–7.
53. Gray TR, Eiden RD, Leonard KE, et al. Identifying prenatal cannabis exposure and effects of concurrent tobacco exposure on neonatal growth. Clin Chem 2010;56: 1442–50.
54. Olsen GD. Placental permeability for drugs of abuse and their metabolites. NIDA Res Monogr 1995;154:152–62.
55. Szeto HH. Kinetics of drug transfer to the fetus. Clin Obstet Gynecol 1993;36: 246–54.
56. Stolk LM, Coenradie SM, Smit BJ, et al. Analysis of methadone and its primary metabolite in meconium. J Anal Toxicol 1997;21:154–9.
57. Jansson LM, Velez M, Harrow C. The opioid-exposed newborn: assessment and pharmacologic management. J Opioid Manag 2009;5:47–55.
58. Sarkar S, Donn SM. Management of neonatal abstinence syndrome in neonatal intensive care units: a national survey. J Perinatol 2006;26:15–7.
59. Kraft WK, Gibson E, Dysart K, et al. Sublingual buprenorphine for treatment of neonatal abstinence syndrome: a randomized trial. Pediatrics 2008;122:601–7.
60. Esmaeili A, Keinhorst AK, Schuster T, et al. Treatment of neonatal abstinence syndrome with clonidine and chloral hydrate. Acta Paediatr 2010;99:209–14.
61. Vearrier D, Greenberg MI, Miller SN, et al. Methamphetamine: history, pathophysiology, adverse health effects, current trends, and hazards associated with the clandestine manufacture of methamphetamine. Dis Mon 2012;58:38–89.
62. Good MM, Solt I, Acuna JG, et al. Methamphetamine use during pregnancy: maternal and neonatal implications. Obstet Gynecol 2010;116:330–4.
63. Yee LM, Wu D. False-positive amphetamine toxicology screen results in three pregnant women using labetalol. Obstet Gynecol 2011;117:503–6.
64. Shakleya DM, Plumley AE, Kraner JC, et al. Trace evidence of trans-phenylpropene as a marker of smoked methamphetamine. J Anal Toxicol 2008;32:705–8.
65. Ladhani NN, Shah PS, Murphy KE. Prenatal amphetamine exposure and birth outcomes: a systematic review and metaanalysis. Am J Obstet Gynecol 2011;205: 219, e1–7.
66. Gareri J, Klein J, Koren G. Drugs of abuse testing in meconium. Clin Chim Acta 2006;366:101–11.
67. Best CA, Laposata M. Fatty acid ethyl esters: toxic non-oxidative metabolites of ethanol and markers of ethanol intake. Front Biosci 2003;8:e202–17.
68. Laposata M. Fatty acid ethyl esters: ethanol metabolites which mediate ethanol-induced organ damage and serve as markers of ethanol intake. Prog Lipid Res 1998;37:307–16.
69. Riley EP, Infante MA, Warren KR. Fetal alcohol spectrum disorders: an overview. Neuropsychol Rev 2011;21:73–80.

Toxicology Testing in Alternative Specimen Matrices

Donald L. Frederick, PhD

KEYWORDS

- Gastric contents • Saliva • Hair • Meconium • Cord blood

KEY POINTS

- Reasons for the use of alternative specimen matrices in toxicology testing include pharmacologic and pharmacokinetic considerations as well as potential ease of collection and availability.
- Gastric lavage is used in patients (frequently pediatric) who have ingested a documented life-threatening amount of poison; specimen must be obtained within 1 hour of ingestion.
- Oral fluid collected from the mouth with or without stimulation is noninvasive and easy to collect, particularly in children, older patients, and chronic disease patients.
- Hair has been used as a specimen relatively little in clinical toxicology testing for metals and drugs but has found use in drug rehabilitation programs.
- In neonatal drug testing, alternative specimens have a significant role in defining what exposure has occurred.

INTRODUCTION

The vast amount of toxicology testing performed in clinical laboratories involves the use of serum, blood, or urine as the specimen. Although blood is often used as a surrogate for measurement of a drug at the site of action, it may not actually represent the concentration at the sites of action. Specific site of action of drugs varies from nerve endings to receptors on cells located throughout the body. Because sampling from these sites is not usually available, blood is used as a monitoring specimen. The rationale is that blood is usually the carrier of the drug from the point of absorption to the site of action. Because most of the drugs are water-soluble, the plasma or serum is a logical source to monitor without the interference of red cells. There are, however, occasions where other types of specimens may be tested, and in some cases may even be required, to obtain the desired clinical information. Most of this testing has only been possible in recent years as a result of the increased sensitivity of the newer

The author has nothing to disclose.
Pathology Department, Peoria Tazewell Pathology Group, 221 NE Glen Oak Avenue, Peoria, IL 61636, USA
E-mail address: dfredpeoria@gmail.com

Clin Lab Med 32 (2012) 467–492
http://dx.doi.org/10.1016/j.cll.2012.06.009
0272-2712/12/$ – see front matter © 2012 Elsevier Inc. All rights reserved.

instrumentation. Many of these alternative specimens have very low concentrations of the drugs, drug metabolites, or other toxins that could not be detected with older techniques. Particularly in the drug field, liquid chromatography–tandem mass spectrometry (LC-MS/MS) has been an analytical tool that has opened the door for testing of alternative specimens. This review looks at these specimens but does not include analysis for infectious diseases, which is another reason for analysis of alternative specimen matrices.

REASONS FOR TESTING

One of the first questions that must be addressed when selecting specimens for testing is "Why." What type of information can be achieved from the specimen selection? Some general questions are

- What is the drug concentration at the site of action?
- What is the drug's metabolic profile?
- What is the patient's exposure to the drug? Is the use recent or long-term?
- What drug exposure is a fetus or newborn likely to have?
- What is the possibility of genotoxic effects?

Pharmacologic Reasons

Historically, one of the additional specimens that was tested was saliva to obtain the "free" portion of a therapeutic drug or hormone. Using saliva free drug concentrations better reflected the amount of drug that could bind to the active site or receptor. Saliva has now become known as oral fluid because the specimen is really a mixture of saliva and other fluids. Alternative specimens are often used for testing of drugs of abuse and in the testing for therapeutic drug management. Earliest uses of saliva were for free drug monitoring such as phenytoin, primidone, and ethosuximide.[1]

Pharmacokinetic Reasons

Various specimens represent differences in the time course that a drug follows in the body. Obviously, for drugs blood is the specimen that reflects the amount of drug that gets circulated throughout the body and is a good approximation of the time when the drug reaches the site of action. To measure duration of action, urine measurements may help in defining the elimination parameters. Other specimens (saliva, sweat, hair, nails, and so forth) may provide specific site of action concentrations or metabolism information for some drugs.

Availability of Specimens

Often in clinical toxicology the case circumstances limit the type of specimens that are available. For a recent ingestion gastric contents may be the best specimen to identify recent oral ingestions, but the specimen may not be easily available because of treatment or patient condition limitations. Patient conditions may also limit the ability to obtain a urine specimen.

Ease of Collection

Alternative specimens such as hair, saliva, and sweat are noninvasive specimens where collections are easily performed with nonskilled collection personnel. Specimens collected in this manner are used in situations in which patient or subject approval may be easier to obtain. Several recent examples include biomonitoring and family toxicology studies.

GASTRIC CONTENTS
Historical Context

Initial evaluation of persons suspected of drug overdose focuses on the signs and symptoms and compares these with some common toxidromes. Historically the first step in the treatment process was to decontaminate the gut starting with gastric lavage. When toxicology laboratories were present in most hospitals, the fluid obtained from the procedure was sent to the laboratory as a stat request, and within a few hours the analysis would define the drug contents of the fluids. The techniques did not have to be very sophisticated because the drugs causing the toxicity were usually high in concentration and without the process of metabolism to confuse the issues. However, over the last decades the toxicology laboratories have all but disappeared, and studies have shown that for most poisoned patients there was not a favorable risk-benefit analysis for decontamination. Gastric fluids if available are still good specimens in limited cases and may offer easy answers for recent oral ingestions.

Physiology

For recent oral ingestions the partially dissolved pills may be present for easy analysis. This scenario most often occurs in pediatric patients where a witness observes the child eat medicines within reach of children. Gastric lavage is reserved for patients who have ingested a documented life-threatening amount of poison. The time period usually is limited to the first hour after ingestion with the exception of drugs that are known to slow gastric emptying and gastrointestinal motility.

Analytes

All pharmaceutical preparations and toxins have at one time or other been detected in gastric fluids following an overdose or toxic exposure. For some emergency department presentations gastric evaluations are still helpful. Other than normal pharmaceuticals, toxins such as amanitin, if detected rapidly in gastric contents, can alter clinical treatment.

ORAL FLUID TESTING
Historical Context

Oral fluid testing has been around for at least 70 years. Dr Langman in a recent review[2] noted that the first look at testing saliva was in 1932, but it was not until the 1970s that drug measurements for therapeutic drug monitoring was begun. The terminology has changed over the years, initially using the term *saliva,* but as the source of the saliva has become known, the more correct term is *oral fluids.*[3] The term *oral fluid* is applied to fluids that are collected from the mouth and may be collected with or without stimulation. The advantages of collecting oral fluid are ease of collection and the noninvasive nature of the collection, particularly in children, older patients, and patients with chronic diseases. Additionally, nonmedical persons can perform collections. These collections can be performed at remote locations where no medical facilities are available. The use of oral fluid in toxicology has been limited by the lack of correlation of drug concentrations between blood and oral fluids and the technology to detect small amounts of drug in limited specimen quantity. With the advent of new highly sensitive technologies, oral fluid has again gained more popularity and use in many aspects of toxicology testing. The major disadvantages of oral fluid specimens are related to contamination of specimens from habits such as smoking or snorting and oral food contamination.

Oral Fluid Physiology

The majority of oral fluid originates from three pairs of major salivary glands with less contribution from minor salivary glands and the gingival crevicular sulci. The fluid collected from the mouth will have bacteria, epithelial cells, erythrocytes, leukocytes, and food debris. This area has been reviewed by Aps and Martens[4] and others.[5,6] Under healthy conditions a person will produce 0 to 6 mL/min of saliva, which should allow for sufficient collection in a reasonable amount of time. The volume and content of saliva produced by the glands varies significantly under autonomic system stimulation and can be stimulated with various external conditions. Acid (citric) stimulation has been used to increase the flow for collection; however, at increased flow rates the pH of the fluid changes, thus the partition coefficient between blood and saliva will change. Depending on the pK_a of the drug, the pH changes will change the drug concentration in the oral fluid collection. Additionally, many therapeutic drugs directly affect the flow of saliva.[4]

Correlation of Plasma Drug Concentrations and Oral Fluid Concentrations

Historically the first use of oral fluids was to measure drug concentrations that were thought to parallel the free drug concentration in plasma. The initial mechanism thought to be involved in the oral fluid drug concentration was a simple filtration of the plasma or diffusion of the free drug concentration from the plasma to the oral fluid, setting up equilibrium and a direct correlation. Whereas this correlation seems to be the result with some drugs, more complex relationships of active excretion and active transport are responsible for the oral fluid concentrations for many more drugs. To determine the relationship between oral fluid concentration and plasma concentration of drugs, various studies have been performed including the correlation of oral fluid concentrations to dose administered. Because of the relative acidity of oral fluid as compared with plasma, basic drugs are frequently found in higher concentrations in the saliva yielding saliva/plasma ratios greater than 1. In early studies with codeine after oral administration, codeine peak plasma levels were observed at 30 minutes to 2 hours. Codeine concentrations in parallel oral fluid collections were significantly elevated, indicating the mouth was contaminated by the oral dose. Investigators estimated that this contamination lasted for 1 hour.[7] The example of lithium where the saliva/plasma ratio is more than 2 indicates that there is an active secretary mechanism or ion trapping that elevates lithium in oral fluid.[2] There are many examples of drugs that have a wide range of plasma to saliva ratios.[8] The fluoro-quinolones have ratios that range from .014 to 1.497 within the same drug class.[9] A general disadvantage of oral fluid specimen is the lack of the presence of phase II metabolites. Glucuronide or sulfate conjugates formed in the liver are rapidly excreted in the urine, and thus no measureable levels are found in the saliva.[10] Because oral fluid specimens are easy to collect, the use of oral specimens in pediatric patients would be ideal. However, in a study looking at morphine, investigators at the Hospital for Sick Children found there was a lack of correlation between saliva and plasma levels.[11]

Another approach to determining the relationship between oral fluids and plasma/blood concentrations is the data provided by studies where simultaneous oral fluid and blood specimens have been analyzed. Because oral fluid specimens have been used in the study of driving impairment, several studies have been published as part of the validation of these procedures.[9,12] In a therapeutic drug study with lamotrigine there was good correlation between oral fluid and serum concentrations, and the investigators support using oral fluid monitoring.[13]

Collection of Oral Fluid Specimens

Collection of saliva can be accomplished by various methods. For research on saliva fluids, individual saliva ducts can be collected by a variety of mechanical aids. For most of the oral fluid collections involved in studies discussed in this review, collection occurs by either spitting into a tube or collection by a pad device. As noted earlier, this collection can be with or without acid stimulation. Once collected, the saliva is usually stored with a buffer to control pH, which will provide a stable environment for screening techniques.

One of the advantages of the use of oral fluids is the ease of collection, but there are hazards associated with collection. Probably the foremost is the issue of contamination. Other issues with collection are effects of stimulation, effects of collection devices, and drug stability with storage. Oral fluid contamination has been demonstrated with cocaine, delta-9-tetrahydrocannibinol (THC), heroin, and codeine.[14] There have been several reviews of oral fluid collection devices, and results indicate that they are not all equivalent.[15–17] There is difference in the amount of oral fluid that can be retrieved from the collection device ranging between 50% to 90% in one study. Recovery of the drugs from the devices was even more variable, ranging from 12% to 98% depending on the drug and device. THC had the worst recoveries, ranging from 12% to 53%. In another study the researchers looked at point of care devices that compared the analysis cutoff with the amount of drug placed into the device.[16] Their results indicate that there is much variability between devices and drug classes.

Recently the collection devices have been combined with a testing device, creating an all-in-one point of care device. Although originally used in roadside surveys of drivers, these devices are being used in drug treatment centers and soon will be available in clinical situations. Dr Verstraete and others have evaluated four of these devices available in 2012.[18] As with previous studies, there is wide variability between testing devices in the four drug classes (amphetamine, THC, cocaine, and morphine) evaluated. Only one of the four devices was able to have greater than 50% sensitivity for all classes, although the specificity for all the devices was high.

Purpose of Oral Fluid Measurements

There are many reasons why oral fluid measurements have found use in clinical practice. Most of the initial studies have focused on the use of oral fluids for the management of therapeutic drug doses. This focus has been expanded to investigate the pharmacokinetic profiles of drugs and use of specific drugs to identify the pharmacogenomics of individuals. As a subset of the therapeutic drug monitoring (TDM) studies, physicians monitoring the drugs used by acute and chronic pain patients have found oral fluids a possible specimen choice. Traditional emergency toxicology has also found some use for oral fluid as a specimen choice. Often this specialty involves drugs of abuse testing, although this method has found more use in the workplace drug testing programs. A related field is the monitoring of exposure to specific drugs such as ethanol and nicotine as part of a wellness program, a rehabilitation program, or a population survey. As a small subset of drug testing, population surveys have found the use of oral fluid as a convenient specimen when large numbers of specimens need to be collected from a variety of locations.

Therapeutic Drug Management

Since the early description of saliva testing for therapeutic drug monitoring was published in 1977,[1,19] many papers have been published on the use of oral fluids for managing drug dosing. One of the limitations of oral fluid testing in TDM is the changing pH of the oral fluids depending on flow rate. The use of oral fluids for the monitoring of anticonvulsants has been well-studied.[20] The use of oral fluid from monitoring phenytoin is particularly attractive because the free phenytoin plasma/saliva ratio has low variability. Monitoring of monotherapy was always more reliable because of drug interactions with saliva flow rate or direct changes on pH of saliva by other drugs such as valproic acid.

Oral fluid monitoring of the newer anticonvulsants may be appropriate. Levetiracetam and topiramate exhibit good correlation between plasma and saliva concentrations.[21,22] Lamotrigine is reported to also have good correlation between salivary and serum concentrations.[13] Oxcarbazepine pharmacologic effect is due to its 10-hydroxy metabolite, and oral fluid can be monitored for this active metabolite.[23] Because the active metabolite is produced in the liver, the oral fluid collection must occur 8 hours after the last dose of oxcarbazepine to allow for conversion and distribution of the metabolite. One use of oral fluid testing that has been studied in connection with anticonvulsants is the home collection of specimens by the patient and shipment via the postal system to the laboratory. Investigators from the University of Kentucky[24] studied the stability of lamotrigine, levetiracetam, oxcarbazepine, topiramate, and zonisamide in oral fluids shipped through the postal system. They found that the stability was sufficient to have dependable monitoring.

Although some benzodiazepines are useful in treatment of epilepsy, routine monitoring of them has not been pursued. Oral fluid testing for benzodiazepines has been used for monitoring of exposure to benzodiazepines such as in workplace testing or drugs of abuse testing. An example where stimulated oral fluid can be used is with bronchodilators. Theophylline has been studied in oral fluid since the 1980s[25–27] and continues to be of value.[28]

Oral fluid testing of other drugs and drug classes has been studied for applicability of therapeutic drug monitoring with limited success. These studies with antipyretic and analgesic drugs, antineoplastic agents, psychoactive drugs, and antiarrhythmics have recently been reviewed.[2,29,30]

Ethanol in oral fluids has been studied since 1938.[2] Ethanol in oral fluids is particularly useful because the saliva measurements were found to parallel capillary blood more closely than the venous blood concentrations.[31] Ethanol breath testing has been more popular and easier to obtain than oral fluid testing. More recently, however, new saliva procedures for ethanol metabolites have been developed. Ethyl glucuronide was one of the first of these; however, the detection time was only a few hours longer than for ethanol, and therefore it is of limited value.[32]

Pharmacokinetic Studies

There have been many investigations over the years into the use of oral fluids in pharmacokinetic evaluations of drug metabolism.[17,33] A later review added studies of gamma-hydroxybutyric acid (GHB), THC, methamphetamine, and 3,4-methylene-dioxymethamphetamine.[34] With the later four drugs, inadequate correlation between oral fluid and plasma specimens caused the investigators to conclude that oral fluid is not an adequate specimen to conduct pharmacokinetic studies.[35,36]

Pharmacogenomics Studies

As personalized medicine becomes more a reality, tests have been developed to ascertain an individualized cytochrome P450 phenotype as an adjunct to knowing the genotype. Probe drugs have been developed where plasma measurement after an oral test dose will reveal the phenotype. An LC-MS/MS method for analysis of dextromethorphan and the O-demethylated metabolite in oral fluid has been developed to ascertain the CYP2D6 individual phenotype.[37] Oral fluid measurements gave data for classification of "poor metabolizers" from "extensive metabolizers." These investigators also provided urine data to give additional information on N-demethylation and glucuronidation, which are not available with the oral fluid data. Another example of this type of study using oral fluids is the use of midazolam to phenotype CYP3A status.

Pain Management Patients

Chronic pain is the leading cause of physician visits, and with the vast array of new drugs or drug combinations used to treat patients the issue of managing these patients and their drug use has become big business.[38] Heltsley and colleagues[38] have compiled over 6441 screening and confirmation results using oral fluids as the specimen. The study found over 40 drug/metabolites originating from 14 drug classes. Their results from these data indicated that there was an 82.7% positive rate with better than 98% positive confirmation rate for the oral fluid screening tests (enzyme-linked immunosorbent assays, ELISAs). The conclusions of these investigators is that oral fluid can be used for the assessment of patients in pain management programs where there is a need to check for their compliance with program guidelines. An interesting finding in the study was that the presence of the N-desalkyl metabolites of buprenorphine, carisoprodol, fentanyl, hydrocodone, methadone, oxycodone, propoxyphene, and tramadol indicated the patient consumed the parent drug and thus these metabolites can be considered biomarkers.[38]

In a recent study investigators analyzed paired urine and oral fluid specimens in 133 paired specimens.[39] This study included analysis for 42 drugs and/or metabolites. There was only a 15% discordant rate between the pairs. One of the major factors in discordant specimen pairs is the kinetic parameters of the drugs between the two fluids: either early appearance in oral fluid prior to excretion or longer excretion pattern in urine as compared with oral fluid. In a study of methadone monitoring, the investigators concluded that the variation in oral fluid pH contributed to the lack of correlation between plasma and oral fluid, and other than obtaining a negative or positive answer, oral fluid for methadone was not a good replacement for plasma monitoring.[40] Although there is not an exact equivalence between oral fluid and urine, oral fluid is useful in evaluation of patients in pain management programs.[41,42] Oral fluid has also been used with newer pain management drugs such as tapentadol.[43]

Emergency Toxicology

Although oral fluid is not the most widely used specimen for clinical toxicology testing, some studies on it have been reported for a variety of drugs. Ethanol was one of the first drugs for saliva testing usually applied to impairment testing, but saliva testing is also used in the physician office setting and emergency departments. In one study, saliva ethanol paralleled blood ethanol more closely than venous sampling.[31] Numerous rapid screening tests have been available as point of care testing devices that emergency departments have used for rapid testing. Most of the devices are for drugs of abuse, but other drugs that have significant abuse potential or significant clinical sequelae are becoming available. For some poisonings urine specimens may be difficult to obtain, and oral fluid may be obtained by nonmedical personnel. Researchers have investigated the use of oral fluid in paraquat poisoning and present two case histories where oral fluid was analyzed with success.[44]

Drugs of Abuse Testing

Oral fluid has become a specimen for testing for use of drugs of abuse within the last 15 years. The distinctive characteristics that make this specimen particularly useful for this type of testing are the ease of collection and less chance for adulteration or substitution of the specimen. Although the use of oral fluids for drug detection is primarily for employment drug testing, oral fluids are used for all areas of performance testing, particularly in drugs and driving cases. Oral fluid testing for drugs of abuse has followed urine drug testing in many aspects including their use of screening tests followed by confirmation testing. As with urine drugs of abuse testing, oral fluid testing has applied cutoffs to each assay to make a call negative or positive. The development of cutoff concentrations has gone through numerous variations, and as in urine drug testing depends on the population being tested and the use of the results. The US federal program from the Department of Health and Human Services has proposed a set of cutoffs for oral fluid tests under their programs. Several other cutoffs have been proposed for other programs. One of the first of these was in the area of driving impairment as under the European Union Roadside Testing–2 (ROSITA-2) program in urine.[45] Because manufacturers follow the areas where there are greatest sales of their products, the cutoffs set by national programs where the numbers of tests are high drive the selection of cutoffs available in the commercial market for screening devices. This tendency is particularly true for testing that is performed in emergency departments or physician offices where simple point of care devices are desired.

Opiates

As part of the new oral fluid screening under Substance Abuse and Mental Health Services Administration (SAMHSA) guidelines, opiate's cutoff was developed as a derivative of the urine program with a lack of controlled dosing studies. Reports from studies of authentic opiate users indicate the proposed cutoffs of 40 μg/L for codeine and morphine, with a 4 μg/L cutoff for 6-acetylmorphine (6-AM) that can be achieved in oral fluids.[46]

Ethanol

The most common specimen to analyze for ethanol is breath, with many standards for clinical as well as forensic breath ethanol analysis. In an attempt to increase the window for which ethanol consumption can be detected, various biomarkers of ethanol have been studied in oral fluid. Ethyl glucuronide (EtG) has been studied with volunteers on different doses of ethanol.[32] Their conclusion was that EtG has only a slightly longer half-life than ethanol in oral fluid.

Nicotine

Nicotine biomarkers are of particular concern to employers and rehabilitation programs to monitor the subject's use of tobacco. The monitoring may be part of a program to monitor compliance on the use of nicotine transdermal medications. In 2010, ELISA screening and LC-MS/MS confirmation of cotinine was studied as related to patient compliance with a transdermal nicotine patch application.[47] In a 2011 study, a wider array of nicotine metabolites were reviewed and compared with known smoking histories.[48,49] Of the metabolites studied in oral fluid, hydroxy-cotinine was slightly better than cotinine for distinguishing smokers from nonsmokers. Investigators also reported that oral fluid nicotine, cotinine, and nicotine/cotinine ratios are applicable for determining smoking exposure in random spot samples.

Other markers of smoking have been tested in oral fluids. Cyanide and thiocyanate measurement in oral fluid has been used mostly to define populations into smokers versus nonsmokers.[50] However, the analysis if readily available may be used for other conditions where elevated cyanide concentrations may be expected.

Cannabinoids and cannabis

THC use, either from smoking, ingestion, or other routes of administration, will result in measureable levels of THC, THC acid, cannabidiol, and cannabinol in oral fluids.[51] Positive results for THC and the acid metabolite were found at 15 minutes after the start of smoking and remained positive for at least 6 hours. Two out of the 6 participants were still positive at 22 hours post dose. The newer "synthetic" cannabinoids are also detected in oral fluid.[51,52]

Benzodiazepines

Benzodiazepines are among the most widely prescribed medications and therefore are among the most abused. With the use of LC-MS/MS technologies, monitoring of a wide variety of benzodiazepines in oral fluid is possible.[53-56]

Amphetamines

As a class of drugs, amphetamines continue to have wide abuse. As one of the original drug classes to be included in the SAMHSA program, amphetamines have proposed cutoffs applied to oral fluids. With an average efficiency of over 85%, amphetamines may accurately be quantitated using the Quantisal collection device and LC-MS/MS methods.[57]

Gamma-hydroxybutyrate

GHB has been studied in connection with forensic cases involving drug facilitated sexual assault and as a party drug. Oral fluid as a specimen for emergency department use would be an ideal solution for patient presentations where a suspected adulterated drink was administered. Rapid procedures have been developed for detection of GHB in oral fluid.[58] Controlled studies reported in 2007 indicate that because GHB is present in oral fluids in concentrations less than that of plasma, oral fluid and sweat are not suitable specimens for monitoring or detecting GHB use.[59]

Metal Testing

Exposure to lead has been a major public health issue.[60,61] All types of specimens including blood, urine, hair, and saliva have been used to evaluate lead exposure in populations and individual patients.[62] Oral fluid has been investigated as a mechanism to monitor populations.[63] Animal studies have shown that saliva can be used to detect lead after a recent exposure and that saliva correlates with plasma lead levels.[64-66] One interesting fact is that essential metal ions are actively transported into salvia rather than passive diffusion. This active transport results in a lack of association with plasma levels, which presents a problem in defining toxic levels in oral fluids. Oral fluid, however, may be more indicative of exposure especially at low levels.[67]

Population Surveys

Oral fluid specimens have a particular attraction for population studies where large numbers of specimens need to be collected at a wide variety of sites. One example of this type of testing is monitoring of arsenic exposure in children playing on playgrounds constructed with copper arsenate–treated wood.[68] In other studies with arsenic there was good correlation between arsenic levels found in oral fluids with the levels found in the drinking water.[69] Other metals including cadmium, chromium, manganese, nickel, and beryllium have either been measured in saliva or proposed to be measured as a method of monitoring exposed populations for metal toxicity.[67,70,71] Another area where oral fluid has been helpful in toxicology is the population studies looking at cotinine and nicotine. Monitoring may be done for a variety of reasons such as secondhand smoking exposure, health evaluations, and population studies.[72]

Testing Methods

There are two schemes for testing of oral fluids. The first scheme mimics the urine drug testing programs where immunoassays are used as screening tests followed by a confirmation test that is usually LC-MS/MS. Because there is very little sample volume with most oral fluid collections, some laboratories have gone directly to LC-MS/MS for screening. In a procedure described in 2007, the investigators were able to screen for 32 drugs in one assay.[73] These investigators used the Intercept device and found less than 50% loss of THC added to the device but acceptable performance of the other drugs. A wide variety of testing schemes have been tried as reviewed in the ROSITA-2 project.[74]

Immunoassay

Immunoassay testing using ELISA has been developed for many drugs and drug metabolites in an oral fluid matrix. A recent list has been published listing 14 essays.[38] Many other evaluations have been performed over the last several years, too numerous to site in this review.[75–78] For physician office or emergency department, point of care devices are available and have been reviewed by several investigators.[34]

The saliva alcohol test is approved by both Clinical Laboratory Improvement Amendments and Department of Transportation as a screening test with sensitivity of .02 g/dL. One device will read semiquantitative answers from .0 to .145 g/dL.

Confirmation testing

The most common method for confirmation of drugs in oral fluid is some version of liquid chromatography mass spectrometry (LC MS). LC-MS/MS is one of the more useful techniques to obtain the needed sensitivity and specificity required for accurate oral fluid testing.[79] Recent methods have been published for a variety of specific drugs.[38] These investigators report their experience in performing over 6400 oral fluid specimens. Another method that is used in a more limited approach for toxicology testing is capillary electrophoresis (CE). CE is coupled with MS for drug detection or as isotachophoresis for ion detection[80] because, like other specimen types, method development is by drug class. Some specific reviews are helpful in evaluating confirmation methods.

Amphetamines

The class of drugs associated with amphetamine is of particular interest for oral fluid testing. Methods have been reported for confirmation and quantitation of five amphetamine derivatives by Fritch and colleagues in 2009.[81] These investigators report their precision and accuracy as well as the extraction recovery from the Intercept collection device. Patients were tested who were enrolled in an addiction recovery program. The limit of detection for amphetamine drug class was generally 2.5 ng/mL.

Opiates

As with any closely related drugs in a drug class, the confirmation methodology must be fully validated to verify accurate and precise results. In a recent review, Tuyay and colleagues describe a validated method for 12 opiates by LC-MS/MS.[82] The collection device used in this research was the Quantisal device. The method uses more than one multiple reaction monitoring transition to assure accuracy and stable isotopic internal standards for a precise assay. A previous review using LC-atmosphere pressure chemical ionization MS/MS provides a slightly different scheme for many of these compounds.[83]

Benzodiazepines

Benzodiazepines are the most frequently detected prescription drugs found in many studies looking at drugs in drivers. As such, this frequency makes them the target of many detection schemes looking at drivers in many countries around the world. The results of many of these studies have been published including a project in the Netherlands.[56,84] Thirty-three benzodiazepines have been identified by a combination of immunoassays and an LC-MS/MS method.

Interpretation of Results

The interpretation of the results of oral fluid testing is dependent on the reasons for testing. Clearly the physiology of the oral fluid production limits the interpretation possibilities. A comprehensive review of the subject appeared in 2007.[85] In general, oral fluid testing will detect recent drug use and is limited in time frame to what is normally found in blood. As discussed earlier, the use of cutoffs in screening tests limits the interpretation of the oral fluid results both from the screening and confirmation tests. There are clearly several issues that affect interpretation of specific drugs such as passive versus active exposure. This exposure can be either oral or vapor (smoke) exposure. Passive smoke exposure from tobacco and marijuana become issues that are generally resolved using cutoff concentrations high enough to eliminate the passive versus active use of the drug. Oral fluid testing is prone to more errors than urine drug testing for these compounds, especially if oral decontamination procedures are not adequate.[34] As with urine testing, oral fluid testing cannot rule out passive exposure as an interpretation of a positive test for THC or nicotine. Appropriate cutoff concentrations may be used to decrease or nearly eliminate these positives from passive inhalation. Recent research on smoked cannabis reports that the proposed cutoffs from SAMHSA offer adequate detection times but do not protect against the possibility of passive cannabis exposure resulting in a positive test.[51,86] If however both the parent THC and the THC-carboxylic acid metabolite are monitored, passive inhalation can be avoided using the appropriate ratios.[87] Continuing research is attempting to define these appropriate levels.[88] For nicotine, the use of cotinine as the test target helps eliminate the contamination issue from the tobacco smoke, and appropriate cutoffs can classify smokers into light or heavy use.[85] Oral fluid has an advantage for the detection of heroin use because the 6-AM/morphine rations are greater than 1.

One clear limitation in the interpretation of any oral fluid test is the collection method and device as cited in the collection section of this article. The changing pH of oral fluid changes the dynamic concentration of drug present, thus limiting the interpretation.[89] Because the use of oral fluid testing for drugs of abuse and other compounds is a new science, there remain limitations on the current research available, and the interpretation of specific results will depend on the data discovered. One area in toxicology where the interpretation of oral fluid tests has been developing rapidly is in roadside testing for driving impairment. As a result of the ROSITA-1 and -2, new technologies are being developed and evaluated to be used in rapid assessment of drug use that can be evaluated against the impairment observed.

HAIR TESTING
Historical Context

One of the first uses of hair analysis was for evaluation of toxic metal exposure. Hair as a specimen provided a window into an extended period of time that was not available by sampling urine or blood. The main disadvantage of hair as a specimen for metal testing is the issue of contamination. Metals and drugs can be adsorbed into the hair in a mechanism where it is difficult to distinguish the amount contributed by external contamination versus the amount that was incorporated into the hair from the body. This contamination aspect is especially true for metals, because environmental dust contains many of the toxic metals that are the subject of monitoring. The interindividual variation in absorption of metals into hair also decreases the accuracy of interpretation.[90] Many metals have been tested from hair of individuals who lived hundreds and even thousands of years ago as part of forensic or historical evaluations.[91] Although metals such as arsenic may be incorporated from the environment, measurement in hair may be an aid in toxicology evaluation of environmental exposure, even if it is not a direct correlation to the current toxic state of the individual. Since 1979 when Baumgartner and colleagues[92] reported finding morphine in hair of heroin abusers, there have been many studies that have shown that other drugs are incorporated into the hair following an individual's drug use.[93,94] There have also been many studies showing that environmental exposure occurs with drugs as it does for metals. In a recent review the investigators found that THC is incorporated from passive smoking.[95]

Hair testing has been used in forensic toxicology and in workplace drug testing but not very often in clinical toxicology. Cone and Preston have published several studies where hair testing has been used a part of heroin treatment programs.[96] Others have published on the use of hair for treatment programs for other drug use such as cocaine. Kintz in 1996[97] reviewed the use of hair in clinical toxicology up until that time.

Hair Physiology

Recent summaries of hair biology indicate that the subject is very complex.[94,98,99] Each hair bulb has its own growth cycle of 2 to 8 years occurring in three stages: the growth stage (anagen), the intermediate stage (catagen), and the resting stage (telogen). Because in the human each follicle is independent, the percentage of hair follicles that are in the growth phase during the time of drug use may vary between active growth (drug incorporation), catagen (little drug incorporation), and resting stage, in which any drug use by the individual would not be incorporated into the hair shaft. One of the problems with hair analysis in a clinical setting is that the drug is incorporated into the hair, but the hair does not grow beyond the scalp for collection for about 8 days.

Collection Methods

Possibly the simplest of the specimen types to collect, hair can be collected and stored with no difficulties. The site of the hair collection depends on the type of analysis that is being requested. If the need is to have the most reproducible specimen, collection usually occurs from the crown of the head where growth rates are known and more reproducible than other sites. If the desire is to find a distant time frame, slower growing hair such as pubic hair may be used. Several investigators have reviewed the amounts of drugs found in the various sampling areas.[100] For marijuana, the highest concentrations were found in the slower growing areas such as pubic hair. After site selection, the method of collection is important. Most collections are taken as small bundles of hair (most recommend the diameter of a pencil) cut off as close to the scalp as possible. If however the most recent data are desired, a plucking of the hair to include the root is desired. This collection would be painful and not normally applied. As methodologies have improved, the sample size needed for accurate detection has decreased. The manner of collection will also change the interpretation of results because drug concentration is higher in the hair root.[101]

Test Analytes

Hair specimens have been used for management of patients in a variety of clinical conditions and situations.[97] One situation in which hair may be useful is for monitoring patients who are unable to provide a reliable history of drug use. The use of phencyclidine may mimic psychiatric disturbances and cause admission to psychiatric units. Sramek and colleagues[102] used hair testing to see if drug use may be responsible for or involved in the hospital admission. This premise can be applied to a variety of clinical situations where long-term use of a drug is not reflected in either the blood or urine specimen results.

Ethanol markers are another example of this principle in the use of hair analysis for the monitoring of parents at risk for having children with fetal alcohol spectrum disorder (FASD).[103,104] Current markers for ethanol abuse are fatty acid ethyl esters (FAEE) and EtG. A recent review of the subject has cited cutoffs that they used to document strict abstinence set at .2 ng/mg for FAEE and 7 pg/mg for EtG.[105,106] In other studies where reported ethanol use was compared with hair analysis of these markers, the investigators concluded that FAEE in hair was correlated to reported use or suspicion of use by health practitioner.[107]

Hair can provide a useful specimen to analyze the active and passive exposure to tobacco smoke. Harmful sequelae from smoking have been known to occur in humans of all ages, but the pregnant woman has added concerns about effects on fetus and fetus development. Premature birth, low birth weight, and other problems such as respiratory disease have been associated with maternal smoking. Hair cotinine has become a good marker to study pregnant women and birth outcomes.[108–110] Another toxin to which the pregnant women is very susceptible is methyl mercury, which can effectively be monitored by maternal hair analysis.[111] The use of cocaine during pregnancy has well-documented detrimental effects. In the last 20 years meconium testing has been the most common way to assess cocaine exposure for the neonate. Maternal and fetal hair, however, offer other choices. Although the timing of drug use versus hair accumulation is not totally understood, hair is a promising choice to evaluate maternal drug use as it relates to fetal outcomes.[112]

Hair has been studied from patients on epileptic medications.[113] Much of the data in the literature show significant individual variation limiting the usefulness in evaluating patient compliance. However, hair testing in a clinical setting may offer answers to specific questions that may affect or modify a clinical treatment. An example of this advantage is in evaluation of cardiac problems in adolescent and young adults with cardiac symptoms. Hair testing to disclose use of amphetamines, cocaine, and cannabinoid relative to symptoms can be helpful in diagnosis and treatment.[114]

There are other clinical conditions where the analytes vary over shorter periods of time and a single blood specimen may not be reflective of the chemical state of the individual. This situation seems to be true for monitoring testosterone levels and the need to treat hypogonadal men. Hair testosterone levels seem to be an accurate reflection of gonadal status in men and may be useful for monitoring therapy.[115] Another such example is hair cortisol, which may better reflect long-term cortisol exposure.[116–119]

Testing Methods

The testing procedures for hair have been developed slowly because there have been issues with some priority extraction procedures. Testing methods have followed many of the other specimen types with screening methods using various immunoassays followed by gas chromatography (GC) or LC MS. The real issue with hair specimens is the cleaning of the specimen prior to analysis. Depending on the analyte, these procedures may be elaborate involving sequential washes in various chemicals or buffers. A review of extraction and analysis methods for benzodiazepines was published by Cirimele and Kintz.[120] Extraction usually involves some form of digestion of the hair and solid phase extraction prior to screening or confirmation tests. Recently new reagents have been developed to automate some of the extraction steps and allow standard immunometric methods to be used.[121,122] Most previous assays followed the urine and oral fluid methodologies. The markers for ethanol abuse, the FAEE, are slightly different with analysis directly on GC MS.[123]

Several newer technologies have been introduced into the screening tests to improve the sensitivity needed for hair analysis. Recent evaluation of new sensitive immunoassays have been compared with standard immunoassays and found more sensitive for amphetamines, benzodiazepines, methadone, cocaine, and opiates.[124] Additionally, the screening assays can be skipped and the sample taken directly to a fast LC procedure with time of flight MS.[125] In another approach, investigators used bead-assisted liquid-liquid extraction and negative ion GC-MS/MS to quantitate marijuana metabolites in hair.[126]

Interpretation of Results

Interpretation of hair test results is limited by what is known about hair growth and deposition of drugs or chemicals into hair. For most individuals drugs may be deposited into hair as the hair forms in the dermal papilla cells. Henderson and colleagues examined the disposition of isotopic labeled cocaine into growing hair by analyzing hair segmented to obtain patterns of drug incorporation.[127] For many individuals the relationship was linear and followed the expected pattern where the drug was found in the hair segments that were growing during the drug use. However, there was another group of subjects with whom there was no direct correlation between the time the drug was used to the time the hair was growing. This result adds doubt to any claim that hair segmentation may give a pattern of drug use. These variations of growth rate and drug incorporation were recently studied at the Federal Bureau of Investigation, resulting in their recommendation to wait 8 weeks from the exposure period before attempting to test hair.[128,129] For many years the subject of drug incorporation into growing hair follicles of varying colors has been debated.[130,131] A recent example of this debate is the finding that methamphetamine is incorporated into pigmented hair at a rate of 2 to 10 times that of white hair.[132]

Because the growth rate of the hair is dependent on the site of sample collection, interpretations of positive results will vary with sample site.[100]

One area that has received much attention in the last decade is the use of hair to evaluate drug and toxin exposure of the unborn fetus during development and the effects of this exposure to the neonate and even later effects on the infant or adolescent. Recent studies with the analysis of cocaine in the hair of mothers have documented significant effects on the neonate associated with positive hair.[133,134] Ethanol markers in hair have been extensively studied. The investigators have tried to establish cutoffs that may be related to the amounts consumed and therefore the possibility of producing FASDs in the neonate.[103,107] There was a direct correlation between social worker reports of alcohol use and the results of the hair test for ethanol markers. The Society of Hair Testing has published proposed cutoffs in hair for EtG and FAEE that can be applied to categorize patients into a group suggesting chronic excessive exposure to ethanol. The society claims the FAEE are sensitive to cosmetic treatment but their incorporation into hair is not biased by hair color.[97]

Hair testing has been a method to look at long-term drug use as it relates to medical procedures other than pregnancy. There is a wide range of procedures where long term-drug use may pose an increased risk of complications or failures of the procedures. One procedure is the assisted reproductive technology wherein drug use may lead to failures and potential poorer outcomes of children conceived.[135]

Hair has been used as the specimen to monitor long-term care. One aspect is the determination of whether appropriate treatment has been given to patients who have limited ability to care for themselves. The findings in these patients often even surprise the attending physician.[136] Sometimes this monitoring can be helpful to determine elderly abuse.[137]

MECONIUM, CORD BLOOD, AND CORD TISSUE
Historical Context

In utero exposure to drugs and other toxins has many consequences for the developing fetus, resulting in immediate developmental issues or latent problems seen only years later. Evaluation of their exposure may include monitoring the mother via a range of specimens and program approaches. As discussed earlier, many alternative specimens may be selected as part of this monitoring program. Often monitoring cannot occur until late in the gestational period or in the newborn period. Alternative specimens have a significant role in defining what exposure has occurred and providing some indication of what the consequences are for the neonate.[138] Initially both the mother and neonate were monitored by serum and urine assays. Because the neonate does not have sufficient readily available urine, other specimens were examined. Meconium is the first fecal matter passed by the neonate and provides a large window into prenatal exposure. Although meconium begins formation between the 12th and 16th week of gestation, the meconium reflects mostly the last trimester of drug or toxin exposure from maternal use. Since the 1980s the methodology for drug testing from meconium has been available. Results of this testing have provided valuable information for the treatment and follow-up of neonates. In some cases meconium has not been available or lost during the collection process, so additional specimens have been examined. Cord blood and cord tissue have been examined as possible samples to evaluate drug and toxin exposure for the neonate. In some cases cord blood specimens have been taken prior to birth, but most studies look at cord blood collected at the time of delivery. Cord tissue has been examined as a specimen that is available at delivery and represents a much longer period of exposure than cord blood, and in at least one study was equivalent to meconium.[139]

Analytes

Numerous drugs of abuse have been analyzed as part of meconium, cord blood, or cord tissue programs. Methamphetamine and cocaine monitoring in human meconium identified exposed infants that have lower birth weights, decreased gestational age, and smaller head circumference.[140,141]

FASD is a detrimental outcome of maternal ethanol abuse. Because the features of this disorder are only obvious in about 10% of ethanol-affected children, large numbers of children are missed where treatment could be beneficial. With the advent of FAEE testing of meconium, these neonates can be identified and be referred to treatment. In a review of the meconium analysis program in Ontario, the investigators concluded that meconium testing of FAEE identified a fivefold increase in detection of these neonates over previous programs.[142,143]

Testing Methods

The testing methods used for meconium, cord blood, and cord tissue are about the same as other specimen types. Various extraction schemes have been proposed over the last 20 years. As with oral fluid specimens, meconium specimens may be taken directly to LC-MS/MS testing as a screening and confirmation technology.

MISCELLANEOUS SPECIMENS
Breast Milk, Ductal Lavage Fluid, Colostrum

On occasion, breast milk is a specimen that must be analyzed. There is continued interest in breast milk analysis as part of a program on nutritional assessment for monitoring the health of newborns. If a newborn is failing to thrive, nutritional deficits may be the primary reason, but toxicology may become an issue on rare occasions. One of the techniques used for analysis is infrared spectroscopy, which has been developed to provide a more rapid assessment of fat, protein, lactose, and total solids in breast milk.[144] Unfortunately there are no published data evaluating drug interferences with these analyses. Drug testing in breast milk is generally concerned with the availability of drug exposure to neonates as a result of maternal drug use.

Sweat

Sweat is an interesting choice of specimen. Probably the first widely available sweat testing was done to aid in the diagnosis of cystic fibrosis. Sweat is collected after stimulation and for a relatively short period of time, 30 minutes, and testing was for chloride ions. Sweat specimens in the area of toxicology offer a wider range of sampling time than offered by blood, urine, or oral fluids. For longer term monitoring of toxicology exposures, hair and nails provide an exposure window of weeks or months but are limited in the sensitivity for limited exposure. Sweat provides an intermediate window to monitor exposure to drugs and other toxins. Sweat collection via a "sweat patch" provides a noninvasive method to obtain a specimen that represents an individual use of drug over the time period the patch is worn; usually 2 weeks. For a review of the sweat patch construction see review by Kidwell, Holland and Athanaselis.[8] Although there have been many questions regarding contamination and collection timing, the collection of sweat over a period of 2 weeks is a viable method for sampling drug exposure in that time period with a noninvasive method. High sensitivity LC-MS/MS methods have enabled drug and drug metabolites to be reliably identified. For drug testing, the sweat patch has been applied to probation monitoring, rehabilitation patients, and parents seeking child custody. The testing has been applied to prenatal testing of mothers suspected of drug use. Sweat testing in these circumstances has several advantages including the longer window of detection, ease of collection, less embarrassing method of collection, and reduced risk of adulteration. A recent report of monitoring for opiates including methadone indicates that this method was effective in monitoring abstinence or drug relapse in a high-risk population.[145,146]

Ethanol is the most abused drug, and monitoring of ethanol has been reviewed in a wide variety of specimens. The use of sweat testing has been studied in patients from abstinence treatment programs. EtG appears in sweat after ethanol use. The result can be related to the amount of ethanol consumed by using a ratio to sodium ions in the sweat patch.[147,148]

Therapeutic drug monitoring for other drugs has been studied including atomoxetine,[149] buprenorphine,[150,151] and methadone.[145] An additional use of sweat sampling is to examine drug metabolism. Methylphenidate time-release kinetics has been studied using sweat collection over 24-hour period via a patch.[152]

Another variation of the sweat testing is a drug swipe similar to the drug swipes law enforcement personnel use to test the presence of drugs on surfaces. The forensic community has a whole line of these tests that test 25 drug groups with simple color tests. Kintz and collegues[153] used these to collect sweat from drivers for monitoring THC use.

Breath

Breath has been the standard specimen for alcohol analysis for many years, both in forensic and employment testing. Breath is used in several clinical situations such as *Helicobacter pylori* testing and breath hydrogen testing. In the diagnostic tests for *H pylori*, a solution of isotopic labeled urea is ingested orally, and the breath is analyzed for the isotopic labeled carbon dioxide. In a recent study, breath was used to analyze for amphetamine, opening up the possibility that breath drug testing can be performed for a wider variety of drugs and analytes.[154]

Other Body Fluids

Numerous other body fluids are analyzed in clinical laboratories for a variety of purposes. Many of these fluids are analyzed for information about infectious processes. As part of this spectrum, various fluids have been analyzed for antibiotic and antiinflammatory drugs to validate that the drug is reaching the needed site of action in sufficient concentration to complete its pharmacologic activity. Synovial fluid has been analyzed for many biological components in efforts to diagnose and monitor disease. Direct measurement of antiinflammatory drugs has been investigated for many years[155] and has found limited use, mostly in research settings.

Another common fluid analyzed in the clinical laboratory is cerebrospinal fluid (CSF). CSF is a very "clean" fluid for toxicology analysis because the protein content is low and drugs can be extracted with ease. CSF as a specimen for toxicology most often is used to answer the question if enough or too much drug has reached the brain. An example would be anticancer drugs that have intrathecal administration. Methotrexate in various treatment protocols used CSF levels to monitor treatment or assess toxicity.

Dried Blood Spots

Although not technically a different specimen type than blood, dried blood spots have unique characteristics that place them in the group of alternative specimens. The use of dried blood spots has unique advantages over blood as the specimen type. Dried blood spots have been used for newborn screening, targeted case management programs, clinical investigations, and epidemiologic studies. The main advantage of dried blood spots is the stability that allows easy transportation from collection site to central laboratory. The technique has been widely used by states to test neonates for inborn errors of metabolism. A recent improvement of the technique using a two-layer membrane instead of normal filter paper to collect the specimen allows for microfiltration of the red blood cells, which reduces the interference of varying hematocrit in the analysis. This technique was recently demonstrated using guanfacine and a semiautomated LC-MS/MS assay.[156] For a recent review of the use of dried blood spots in toxicology, consult Stove and colleagues.[157] These techniques have been applied to TDM for children.[158,159]

REFERENCES

1. Horning MG, Brown L, Nowlin J, et al. Use of saliva in therapeutic drug monitoring. Clin Chem 1977;23:157–64.
2. Langman LJ. The use of oral fluid for therapeutic drug management: clinical and forensic toxicology. Ann N Y Acad Sci 2007;1098:145–66.
3. Siegel IA. The role of saliva in drug monitoring. Ann N Y Acad Sci 1993;694:86–90.
4. Aps JK, Martens LC. Review: the physiology of saliva and transfer of drugs into saliva. Forensic Sci Int 2005;150:119–31.
5. Farnaud SJ, Kosti O, Getting SJ, et al. Saliva: physiology and diagnostic potential in health and disease. Scientific World Journal 2010;10:434–56.
6. Dawes C. Salivary flow patterns and the health of hard and soft oral tissues. J Am Dent Assoc 2008;139(Suppl):18S–24S.
7. O'Neal CL, Crouch DJ, Rollins DE, et al. Correlation of saliva codeine concentrations with plasma concentrations after oral codeine administration. J Anal Toxicol 1999;23:452–9.
8. Kidwell DA, Holland JC, Athanaselis S. Testing for drugs of abuse in saliva and sweat. J Chromatogr B Biomed Sci Appl 1998;713:111–35.
9. Mullangi R, Agrawal S, Srinivas NR. Measurement of xenobiotics in saliva: is saliva an attractive alternative matrix? Case studies and analytical perspectives. Biomed Chromatogr 2009;23:3–25.
10. Lee HS, Ti TY, Koh YK, et al. Paracetamol elimination in Chinese and Indians in Singapore. Eur J Clin Pharmacol 1992;43:81–4.
11. Kopecky EA, Jacobson S, Klein J, et al. Correlation of morphine sulfate in blood plasma and saliva in pediatric patients. Ther Drug Monit 1997;19:530–4.
12. Wille SM, Raes E, Lillsunde P, et al. Relationship between oral fluid and blood concentrations of drugs of abuse in drivers suspected of driving under the influence of drugs. Ther Drug Monit 2009;31:511–9.
13. Ryan M, Grim SA, Miles MV, et al. Correlation of lamotrigine concentrations between serum and saliva. Pharmacotherapy 2003;23:1550–7.
14. Crouch DJ. Oral fluid collection: the neglected variable in oral fluid testing. Forensic Sci Int 2005;150:165–73.
15. Drummer OH. Introduction and review of collection techniques and applications of drug testing of oral fluid. Ther Drug Monit 2008;30:203–6.

16. Crouch DJ, Walsh JM, Cangianelli L, et al. Laboratory evaluation and field application of roadside oral fluid collectors and drug testing devices. Ther Drug Monit 2008;30: 188–95.
17. Drummer OH. Drug testing in oral fluid. Clin Biochem Rev 2006;27:147–59.
18. Vanstechelman S, Isalberti C, Van der Linden T, et al. Analytical evaluation of four on-site oral fluid drug testing devices. J Anal Toxicol 2012;36:136–40.
19. Dvorchik BH, Vesell ES. Pharmacokinetic interpretation of data gathered during therapeutic drug monitoring. Clin Chem 1976;22:868–78.
20. Liu H, Delgado MR. Therapeutic drug concentration monitoring using saliva samples. Focus on anticonvulsants. Clin Pharmacokinet 1999;36:453–70.
21. Miles MV, Tang PH, Glauser TA, et al. Topiramate concentration in saliva: an alternative to serum monitoring. Pediatr Neurol 2003;29:143–7.
22. Grim SA, Ryan M, Miles MV, et al. Correlation of levetiracetam concentrations between serum and saliva. Ther Drug Monit 2003;2561–6.
23. Miles MV, Tang PH, Ryan MA, et al. Feasibility and limitations of oxcarbazepine monitoring using salivary monohydroxycarbamazepine (MHD). Ther Drug Monit 2004;26:300–4.
24. Jones MD, Ryan M, Miles MV, et al. Stability of salivary concentrations of the newer antiepileptic drugs in the postal system. Ther Drug Monit 2005;27(5):576–9.
25. Jaber M, Schneider AT, Goldstein S, et al. Reliability and predictive value of salivary theophylline levels. Ann Allergy 1987;58:105–8.
26. Blanchard J, Harvey S, Morgan WJ. Relationship between serum and saliva theophylline levels in patients with cystic fibrosis. Ther Drug Monit 1992;14:48–54.
27. Blanchard J, Harvey S, Morgan WJ. Serum/saliva correlations for theophylline in asthmatics. J Clin Pharmacol 1991;31:565–70.
28. Henkin RI. Comparative monitoring of oral theophylline treatment in blood serum, saliva, and nasal mucus. Ther Drug Monit 2012;34:217–21.
29. Maudens KE, Stove CP, Lambert WE. Quantitative liquid chromatographic analysis of anthracyclines in biological fluids. J Chromatogr B Analyt Technol Biomed Life Sci 2011;879:2471–86.
30. Maudens KE, Stove CP, Cocquyt VF, et al. Development and validation of a liquid chromatographic method for the simultaneous determination of four anthracyclines and their respective 13-S-dihydro metabolites in plasma and saliva. J Chromatogr B Analyt Technol Biomed Life Sci 2009;877(30):3907–15.
31. Haeckel R, Bucklitsch I. The comparability of ethanol concentrations in peripheral blood and saliva. The phenomenon of variation in saliva to blood concentration ratios. J Clin Chem Clin Biochem 1987;25:199–204.
32. Hoiseth G, Yttredal B, Karinen R, et al. Ethyl glucuronide concentrations in oral fluid, blood, and urine after volunteers drank 0.5 and 1.0 g/kg doses of ethanol. J Anal Toxicol 2010;34:310–24.
33. Drummer OH. Review: pharmacokinetics of illicit drugs in oral fluid. Forensic Sci Int 2005;150:133–42.
34. Pil K, Verstraete A. Current developments in drug testing in oral fluid. Ther Drug Monit 2008;30:196–202.
35. Link B, Haschke M, Grignaschi N, et al. Pharmacokinetics of intravenous and oral midazolam in plasma and saliva in humans: usefulness of saliva as matrix for CYP3A phenotyping. Br J Clin Pharmacol 2008;66:473–84.
36. Link B, Haschke M, Wenk M, et al. Determination of midazolam and its hydroxy metabolites in human plasma and oral fluid by liquid chromatography/electrospray ionization ion trap tandem mass spectrometry. Rapid Commun Mass Spectrom 2007;21:1531–40.

37. Lutz U, Völkel W, Lutz RW, et al. LC-MS/MS analysis of dextromethorphan metabolism in human saliva and urine to determine CYP2D6 phenotype and individual variability in N-demethylation and glucuronidation. J Chromatogr B Analyt Technol Biomed Life Sci 2004;813:217–25.
38. Heltsley R, DePriest A, Black DL, et al. Oral fluid drug testing of chronic pain patients. I. Positive prevalence rates of licit and illicit drugs. J Anal Toxicol 2011;35:529–40.
39. Heltsley R, DePriest A, Black DL, et al. Oral fluid drug testing of chronic pain patients. II. Comparison of paired oral fluid and urine specimens. J Anal Toxicol 2012;36:75–80.
40. Shiran MR, Hassanzadeh-Khayyat M, Iqbal MZ, et al. Can saliva replace plasma for the monitoring of methadone? Ther Drug Monit 2005;27:580–6.
41. Moore C, Rana S, Coulter C. Determination of meperidine, tramadol and oxycodone in human oral fluid using solid phase extraction and gas chromatography-mass spectrometry. J Chromatogr B Analyt Technol Biomed Life Sci 2007;850:370–5.
42. Coulter C, Taruc M, Tuyay J, et al. Antidepressant drugs in oral fluid using liquid chromatography-tandem mass spectrometry. J Anal Toxicol 2010;34:64–72.
43. Coulter C, Taruc M, Tuyay J, et al. Determination of tapentadol and its metabolite N-desmethyltapentadol in urine and oral fluid using liquid chromatography with tandem mass spectral detection. J Anal Toxicol 2010;34:458–63.
44. Lanaro R, Costa JL, Fernandes LC, et al. Detection of paraquat in oral fluid, plasma, and urine by capillary electrophoresis for diagnosis of acute poisoning. J Anal Toxicol 2011;35:274–9.
45. Verstraete A, Raes E. ROSITA-2 Project final report. Gent (Belgium): Ghent University Department of Clinical Biology, Microbiology and Immunity; 2006. p. 1–257.
46. Garnier M, Coulter C, Moore C. Selection of an immunoassay screening cutoff concentration for opioids in oral fluid. J Anal Toxicol 2011;35:369–74.
47. Miller EI, Norris HR, Rollins DE, et al. Identification and quantification of nicotine biomarkers in human oral fluid from individuals receiving low-dose transdermal nicotine: a preliminary study. J Anal Toxicol 2010;34:357–66.
48. Scheidweiler KB, Shakleya DM, Huestis MA. Simultaneous quantification of nicotine, cotinine, trans-3'-hydroxycotinine, norcotinine and mecamylamine in human urine by liquid chromatography-tandem mass spectrometry. Clin Chim Acta 2012;413:978–84.
49. Scheidweiler KB, Marrone GF, Shakleya DM, et al. Oral fluid nicotine markers to assess smoking status and recency of use. Ther Drug Monit 2011;33:609–18.
50. Paul BD. Smith ML. Cyanide and thiocyanate in human saliva by gas chromatography-mass spectrometry. J Anal Toxicol 2006;30:511–5.
51. Lee D, Schwope DM, Milman G, et al. Cannabinoid disposition in oral fluid after controlled smoked cannabis. Clin Chem 2012;58:748–56.
52. Coulter CM, Garnier M, Moore C. Synthetic cannabinoids in oral fluid. J Anal Toxicol 2011;35:424–30.
53. Blencowe T, Pehrsson A, Lillsunde P, et al. An analytical evaluation of eight on-site oral fluid drug screening devices using laboratory confirmation results from oral fluid. Forensic Sci Int 2011;208:173–9.
54. Gronholm M, Lillsunde P. A comparison between on-site immunoassay drug-testing devices and laboratory results. Forensic Sci Int 2001;121:37–46.
55. Moore C, Coulter C, Crompton K, et al. Determination of benzodiazepines in oral fluid using LC-MS-MS. J Anal Toxicol 2007;31:596–600.
56. Smink BE, Mathijssen MP, Lusthof KJ, et al. Comparison of urine and oral fluid as matrices for screening of thirty-three benzodiazepines and benzodiazepine-like substances using immunoassay and LC-MS(-MS). J Anal Toxicol 2006;30:478–85.

57. Moore C, Coulter C, Crompton K. Achieving proposed federal concentrations using reduced specimen volume for the extraction of amphetamines from oral fluid. J Anal Toxicol 2007;31:442–6.
58. De Paoli G, Bell S. A rapid GC-MS determination of gamma-hydroxybutyrate in saliva. J Anal Toxicol 2008;32:298–302.
59. Abanades S, Farré M, Segura M, et al. Disposition of gamma-hydroxybutyric acid in conventional and nonconventional biologic fluids after single drug administration: issues in methodology and drug monitoring. Ther Drug Monit 2007;29:64–70.
60. Juberg DR, Kleiman CF, Kwon SC. Position paper of the American Council on Science and Health: lead and human health. Ecotoxicol Environ Saf 1997;38:162–80.
61. Keller DA, Juberg DR, Catlin N, et al. Identification and characterization of adverse effects in 21st century toxicology. Toxicol Sci 2012;126:291–7.
62. Pirkle JL, Needham LL, Sexton K. Improving exposure assessment by monitoring human tissues for toxic chemicals. J Expo Anal Environ Epidemiol 1995;5:405–24.
63. Gonzalez M, Banderas JA, Baez A, et al. Salivary lead and cadmium in a young population residing in Mexico City. Toxicol Lett 1997;93:55–64.
64. Timchalk C, Lin Y, Weitz KK, et al. Disposition of lead (Pb) in saliva and blood of Sprague-Dawley rats following a single or repeated oral exposure to Pb-acetate. Toxicology 2006;222:86–94.
65. Yantasee W, Timchalk C, Weitz KK, et al. Optimization of a portable microanalytical system to reduce electrode fouling from proteins associated with biomonitoring of lead (Pb) in saliva. Talanta 2005;67:617–24.
66. Yantasee W, Timchalk C, Lin Y. Microanalyzer for biomonitoring lead (Pb) in blood and urine. Anal Bioanal Chem 2007;387:335–41.
67. Gil F, Hernández AF, Márquez C, et al. Biomonitorization of cadmium, chromium, manganese, nickel and lead in whole blood, urine, axillary hair and saliva in an occupationally exposed population. Sci Total Environ 2011;409:1172–80.
68. Lew K, Acker JP, Gabos S, et al. Biomonitoring of arsenic in urine and saliva of children playing on playgrounds constructed from chromated copper arsenate-treated wood. Environ Sci Technol 2010;44:3986–91.
69. Yuan C, Lu X, Oro N, et al. Arsenic speciation analysis in human saliva. Clin Chem 2008;54:163–71.
70. Olmedo P, Pla A, Hernández AF, et al. Validation of a method to quantify chromium, cadmium, manganese, nickel and lead in human whole blood, urine, saliva and hair samples by electrothermal atomic absorption spectrometry. Anal Chim Acta 2010;659:60–7.
71. Sutton M, Burastero SR. Beryllium chemical speciation in elemental human biological fluids. Chem Res Toxicol 2003;16:1145–54
72. Schutte-Borkovec K, Heppel CW, Heling AK, et al. Analysis of myosmine, cotinine and nicotine in human toenail, plasma and saliva. Biomarkers 2009;14:278–84.
73. Oiestad EL, Johansen U, Christophersen AS. Drug screening of preserved oral fluid by liquid chromatography-tandem mass spectrometry. Clin Chem 2007;53:300–9.
74. Lillsunde P. Analytical techniques for drug detection in oral fluid. Ther Drug Monit 2008;30:181–7.
75. Wille SM, Samyn N, Ramírez-Fernández Mdel M, et al. Evaluation of on-site oral fluid screening using Drugwipe-5(+), RapidSTAT and Drug Test 5000 for the detection of drugs of abuse in drivers. Forensic Sci Int 2010;198:2–6.
76. Jaedicke KM, Taylor JJ, Preshaw PM. Validation and quality control of ELISAs for the use with human saliva samples. J Immunol Methods 2012;377:62–5.

77. Huestis MA, Verstraete A, Kwong TC, et al. Oral fluid testing: promises and pitfalls. Clin Chem 2011;57:805–10.

78. Schwope DM, Milman G, Huestis MA. Validation of an enzyme immunoassay for detection and semiquantification of cannabinoids in oral fluid. Clin Chem 2010;56: 1007–14.

79. Wylie FM, Torrance H, Anderson RA, et al. Drugs in oral fluid Part I. Validation of an analytical procedure for licit and illicit drugs in oral fluid. Forensic Sci Int 2005;150: 191–8.

80. Lloyd DK. Capillary electrophoresis analysis of biofluids with a focus on less commonly analyzed matrices. J Chromatogr B Analyt Technol Biomed Life Sci 2008;866: 154–66.

81. Fritch D, Blum K, Nonnemacher S, et al. Identification and quantitation of amphetamines, cocaine, opiates, and phencyclidine in oral fluid by liquid chromatography-tandem mass spectrometry. J Anal Toxicol 2009;33:569–77.

82. Tuyay J, Coulter C, Rodrigues W, et al. Disposition of opioids in oral fluid: Importance of chromatography and mass spectral transitions in LC-MS/MS. Drug Test Anal 2012;4(6):395–401.

83. Dams R, Murphy CM, Choo RE, et al. LC-atmospheric pressure chemical ionization-MS/MS analysis of multiple illicit drugs, methadone, and their metabolites in oral fluid following protein precipitation. Anal Chem 2003;75:798–804.

84. Smink BE, Egberts AC, Lusthof KJ, et al. The relationship between benzodiazepine use and traffic accidents: A systematic literature review. CNS Drugs 2010;24:639–53.

85. Cone EJ, Huestis MA. Interpretation of oral fluid tests for drugs of abuse. Ann N Y Acad Sci 2007;1098:51–103.

86. Lee D, Schwope DM, Milman G, et al. Oral fluid cannabinoids in chronic, daily Cannabis smokers during sustained, monitored abstinence. Clin Chem 2011;57: 1127–36.

87. Moore C, Coulter C, Uges D, et al. Cannabinoids in oral fluid following passive exposure to marijuana smoke. Forensic Sci Int 2011;212:227–30.

88. Toennes SW, Ramaekers JG, Theunissen EL, et al. Pharmacokinetic properties of delta9-tetrahydrocannabinol in oral fluid of occasional and chronic users. J Anal Toxicol 2010;34:216–21.

89. Kato K, Hillsgrove M, Weinhold L, et al. Cocaine and metabolite excretion in saliva under stimulated and nonstimulated conditions. J Anal Toxicol 1993;17:338–41.

90. Hindmarsh JT. Caveats in hair analysis in chronic arsenic poisoning. Clin Biochem 2002;35:1–11.

91. Egeland GM, Ponce R, Knecht R, et al. Trace metals in ancient hair from the Karluk Archaeological Site, Kodiak, Alaska. Int J Circumpolar Health 1999;58:52–6.

92. Baumgartner AM, Jones PF, Baumgartner WA, et al. Radioimmunoassay of hair for determining opiate-abuse histories. J Nucl Med 1979;20:748–52.

93. Kintz P, Villain M, Cirimele V. Hair analysis for drug detection. Ther Drug Monit 2006;28:442–6.

94. Barroso M, Gallardo E, Vieira DN, et al. Hair: a complementary source of bioanalytical information in forensic toxicology. Bioanalysis 2011;3:67–79.

95. Auwarter V, Wohlfarth A, Traber J, et al. Hair analysis for Delta9-tetrahydrocannabinolic acid A–new insights into the mechanism of drug incorporation of cannabinoids into hair. Forensic Sci Int 2010;196:10–3.

96. Cone EJ, Preston KL. Toxicologic aspects of heroin substitution treatment. Ther Drug Monit 2002;24:193–8.

97. Kintz P, editor. Drug testing in hair. Boca Raton (FL): CRC Press; 1996.

98. Driskell RR, Clavel C, Rendl M, et al. Hair follicle dermal papilla cells at a glance. J Cell Sci 2011;124:1179–82.

99. Shimomura Y, Christiano AM. Biology and genetics of hair. Annu Rev Genomics Hum Genet 2010;11:109–32.

100. Han E, Choi H, Lee S, et al. A comparative study on the concentrations of 11-nor-Delta9-tetrahydrocannabinol-9-carboxylic acid (THCCOOH) in head and pubic hair. Forensic Sci Int 2011;212:238–41.

101. Han E, Choi H, Lee S. A study on the concentrations of 11-nor-Delta(9)-tetrahydro-cannabinol-9-carboxylic acid (THCCOOH) in hair root and whole hair. Forensic Sci Int 2011;210:201–5.

102. Sramek JJ, Baumgartner WA, Tallos JA, et al. Hair analysis for detection of phencyclidine in newly admitted psychiatric patients. Am J Psychiatry 1985;142:950–3.

103. Kulaga V, Shor S, Koren G. Correlation between drugs of abuse and alcohol by hair analysis: parents at risk for having children with fetal alcohol spectrum disorder. Alcohol 2010;44:615–21.

104. Kulaga V, Pragst F, Fulga N, et al. Hair analysis of fatty acid ethyl esters in the detection of excessive drinking in the context of fetal alcohol spectrum disorders. Ther Drug Monit 2009;31:261–6.

105. Pragst F, Rothe M, Moench B, et al. Combined use of fatty acid ethyl esters and ethyl glucuronide in hair for diagnosis of alcohol abuse: interpretation and advantages. Forensic Sci Int 2010;196:101–10.

106. Pragst F, Yegles M. Determination of fatty acid ethyl esters (FAEE) and ethyl glucuronide (EtG) in hair: a promising way for retrospective detection of alcohol abuse during pregnancy? Ther Drug Monit 2008;30:255–63.

107. Kulaga V, Gareri J, Fulga N, et al. Agreement between the fatty acid ethyl ester hair test for alcohol and social workers' reports. Ther Drug Monit 2010;32:294–9.

108. Florescu A, Ferrence R, Einarson T, et al. Methods for quantification of exposure to cigarette smoking and environmental tobacco smoke: focus on developmental toxicology. Ther Drug Monit 2009;31:14–30.

109. Florescu A, Ferrence R, Einarson TR, et al. Reference values for hair cotinine as a biomarker of active and passive smoking in women of reproductive age, pregnant women, children, and neonates: systematic review and meta-analysis. Ther Drug Monit 2007;29:437–46.

110. Klein J, Koren G. Hair analysis–a biological marker for passive smoking in pregnancy and childhood. Hum Exp Toxicol 1999;18:279–82.

111. Cace IB, Milardovic A, Prpic I, et al. Relationship between the prenatal exposure to low-level of mercury and the size of a newborn's cerebellum. Med Hypotheses 2011;76:514–6.

112. Garcia-Bournissen F, Rokach B, Karaskov T, et al. Cocaine detection in maternal and neonatal hair: implications to fetal toxicology. Ther Drug Monit 2007;29:71–6.

113. Williams J, Lawthom C, Dunstan FD, et al. Variability of antiepileptic medication taking behaviour in sudden unexplained death in epilepsy: hair analysis at autopsy. J Neurol Neurosurg Psychiatry 2006;77:481–4.

114. Klys M, Szydlowski L, Rojek S. Role of toxicological determinations of amphet-amines and cannabinoids in hair of adolescent patients in cardiologic diagnostic management. Cardiol Young 2012;22:8–12.

115. Thomson S, Koren G, Van Steen V, et al. Testosterone concentrations in hair of hypogonadal men with and without testosterone replacement therapy. Ther Drug Monit 2009;31:779–82.

116. Gow R, Koren G, Rieder M, Van Uum S. Hair cortisol content in patients with adrenal insufficiency on hydrocortisone replacement therapy. Clin Endocrinol (Oxf) 2011;74: 687–93.

117. Gow R, Thomson S, Rieder M, et al. An assessment of cortisol analysis in hair and its clinical applications. Forensic Sci Int 2010;196:32–7.

118. Russell E, Koren G, Rieder M, et al. Hair cortisol as a biological marker of chronic stress: Current status, future directions and unanswered questions. Psychoneuroendocrinology 2012;37:589–601.

119. Sauve B, Koren G, Walsh G, et al. Measurement of cortisol in human hair as a biomarker of systemic exposure. Clin Invest Med 2007;30:E183–91.

120. Cirimele V, Kintz P. Identification of benzodiazepines in human hair: a review. In: Salamone SJ, editor. Benzodiazepines and GHB: detection and pharmacology. Totowa (NJ): Humana Press; 2001. p. 77–92.

121. de la Torre R, Civit E, Svaizer F, et al. High throughput analysis of drugs of abuse in hair by combining purposely designed sample extraction compatible with immunometric methods used for drug testing in urine. Forensic Sci Int 2010;196:18–21.

122. Baumgartner MR, Guglielmello R, Fanger M, et al. Analysis of drugs of abuse in hair: evaluation of the immunochemical method VMA-T vs. LC-MS/MS or GC-MS. Forensic Sci Int 2012;215:56–9.

123. Zimmermann CM, Jackson GP. Gas chromatography tandem mass spectrometry for biomarkers of alcohol abuse in human hair. Ther Drug Monit 2010;32:216–23.

124. Musshoff F, Kirschbaum KM, Graumann K, et al. Evaluation of two immunoassay procedures for drug testing in hair samples. Forensic Sci Int 2012;215:60–3.

125. Dominguez-Romero JC, Garcia-Reyes JF, Molina-Diaz A. Screening and quantitation of multiclass drugs of abuse and pharmaceuticals in hair by fast liquid chromatography electrospray time-of-flight mass spectrometry. J Chromatogr B Analyt Technol Biomed Life Sci 2011;879:2034–42.

126. Kim JY, Cheong JC, Lee JI, et al. Improved gas chromatography-negative ion chemical ionization tandem mass spectrometric method for determination of 11-nor-Delta9-tetrahydrocannabinol-9-carboxylic acid in hair using mechanical pulverization and bead-assisted liquid-liquid extraction. Forensic Sci Int 2011;206:e99–102.

127. Henderson GL, Harkey MR, Zhou C, et al. Incorporation of isotopically labeled cocaine and metabolites into human hair: 1. Dose-response relationships. J Anal Toxicol 1996;20:1–12.

128. LeBeau MA, Montgomery MA, Brewer JD. The role of variations in growth rate and sample collection on interpreting results of segmental analyses of hair. Forensic Sci Int 2011;210:110–6.

129. LeBeau MA. Guidance for improved detection of drugs used to facilitate crimes. Ther Drug Monit 2008;30:229–33.

130. Joseph RE Jr, Su TP, Cone EJ. In vitro binding studies of drugs to hair: influence of melanin and lipids on cocaine binding to Caucasoid and Africoid hair. J Anal Toxicol 1996;20:338–44.

131. Henderson GL, Harkey MR, Zhou C, et al. Incorporation of isotopically labeled cocaine into human hair: race as a factor. J Anal Toxicol 1998;22:156–65.

132. Han E, Park Y, Kim E, et al. The dependence of the incorporation of methamphetamine into rat hair on dose, frequency of administration and hair pigmentation. J Chromatogr B Analyt Technol Biomed Life Sci 2010;878:2845–51.

133. Falcon M, Pichini S, Joya J, et al. Maternal hair testing for the assessment of fetal exposure to drug of abuse during early pregnancy: comparison with testing in placental and fetal remains. Forensic Sci Int 2011;218:92–6.

134. Joya X, Gomez-Culebras M, Callejón A, et al. Cocaine use during pregnancy assessed by hair analysis in a Canary Islands cohort. BMC Pregnancy Childbirth 2012;12:2.

135. Pichini S, De Luca R, Pellegrini M, et al. Hair and urine testing to assess drugs of abuse consumption in couples undergoing assisted reproductive technology (ART). Forensic Sci Int 2012;218:57–61.

136. Musshoff F, Lachenmeier K, Trafkowski J, et al. Determination of opioid analgesics in hair samples using liquid chromatography/tandem mass spectrometry and application to patients under palliative care. Ther Drug Monit 2007;29:655–61.

137. Kintz P, Villain M, Cirimele V. Chemical abuse in the elderly: evidence from hair analysis. Ther Drug Monit 2008;30:207–11.

138. Lozano J, García-Algar O, Vall O, et al. Biological matrices for the evaluation of in utero exposure to drugs of abuse. Ther Drug Monit 2007;29:711–34.

139. Montgomery D, Plate C, Alder SC, et al. Testing for fetal exposure to illicit drugs using umbilical cord tissue vs meconium. J Perinatol 2006;26:11–4.

140. Gray TR, Kelly T, LaGasse LL, et al. New meconium biomarkers of prenatal methamphetamine exposure increase identification of affected neonates. Clin Chem 2010;56:856–60.

141. Gray TR, Kelly T, LaGasse LL, et al. Novel biomarkers of prenatal methamphetamine exposure in human meconium. Ther Drug Monit 2009;31:70–5.

142. Hutson JR, Rao C, Fulga N, et al. An improved method for rapidly quantifying fatty acid ethyl esters in meconium suitable for prenatal alcohol screening. Alcohol 2011;45:193–9.

143. Gareri J, Lynn H, Handley M, et al. Prevalence of fetal ethanol exposure in a regional population-based sample by meconium analysis of fatty acid ethyl esters. Ther Drug Monit 2008;30:239–45.

144. Casadio YS, Williams TM, Lai CT, et al. Evaluation of a mid-infrared analyzer for the determination of the macronutrient composition of human milk. J Hum Lact 2010; 26:376–83.

145. Barnes AJ, Brunet BR, Choo RE, et al. Excretion of methadone in sweat of pregnant women throughout gestation after controlled methadone administration. Ther Drug Monit 2010;32:497–503.

146. Brunet BR, Barnes AJ, Choo RE, et al. Monitoring pregnant women's illicit opiate and cocaine use with sweat testing. Ther Drug Monit 2010;32:40–9.

147. Appenzeller BM, Schummer C, Rodrigues SB, et al. Determination of the volume of sweat accumulated in a sweat-patch using sodium and potassium as internal reference. J Chromatogr B Analyt Technol Biomed Life Sci 2007;852:333–7.

148. Schummer C, Appenzeller BM, Wennig R. Quantitative determination of ethyl gluouronide in sweat. Ther Drug Monit 2008;30:536–9.

149. Marchei E, Papaseit E, Garcia-Algar OQ, et al. Determination of atomoxetine and its metabolites in conventional and non-conventional biological matrices by liquid chromatography-tandem mass spectrometry. J Pharm Biomed Anal 2012;60: 26–31.

150. Concheiro M, Jones HE, Johnson RE, et al. Preliminary buprenorphine sublingual tablet pharmacokinetic data in plasma, oral fluid, and sweat during treatment of opioid-dependent pregnant women. Ther Drug Monit 2011;33:619–26.

151. Concheiro M, Shakleya DM, Huestis MA. Simultaneous analysis of buprenorphine, methadone, cocaine, oplates and nicotine metabolites in sweat by liquid chromatography tandem mass spectrometry. Anal Bioanal Chem 2011;400:69–78.

152. Marchei E, Farré M, Pardo R, et al. Usefulness of sweat testing for the detection of methylphenidate after fast- and extended-release drug administration: a pilot study. Ther Drug Monit 2010;32:508–11.
153. Kintz P, Cirimele V, Ludes B. Detection of cannabis in oral fluid (saliva) and forehead wipes (sweat) from impaired drivers. J Anal Toxicol 2000;24:557–61.
154. Beck O, Leine K, Palmskog G, et al. Amphetamines detected in exhaled breath from drug addicts: a new possible method for drugs-of-abuse testing. J Anal Toxicol 2010;34: 233–7.
155. Day RO, McLachlan AJ, Graham GG, et al. Pharmacokinetics of nonsteroidal anti-inflammatory drugs in synovial fluid. Clin Pharmacokinet 1999;36:191–210.
156. Li Y, Henion J, Abbott R, et al. The use of a membrane filtration device to form dried plasma spots for the quantitative determination of guanfacine in whole blood. Rapid Commun Mass Spectrom 2012;26:1208–12.
157. Stove CP, Ingels AS, De Kesel PM, et al. Dried blood spots in toxicology: from the cradle to the grave? Crit Rev Toxicol 2012;42:230–43.
158. Pandya HC, Spooner N, Mulla H. Dried blood spots, pharmacokinetic studies and better medicines for children. Bioanalysis 2011;3:779–86.
159. Patel P, Mulla H, Tanna S, et al. Facilitating pharmacokinetic studies in children: a new use of dried blood spots. Arch Dis Child 2010;95:484–7.

Principles and Procedures in Forensic Toxicology

John F. Wyman, PhD

KEYWORDS

- Review • Drugs • Analysis • Forensic • Toxicology • Procedures

KEY POINTS

- Forensic Toxicology is composed of Postmortem Toxicology, Human Performance Toxicology and Drug Urinalysis.
- Forensic Toxicology results have the potential of being scrutinized in court; as a result, testing is more comprehensive, with greater emphasis on specificity and accuracy in identifying potential toxicants.
- Conclusions about postmortem results must be made after considering all aspects of a case, including medical records, matrices analyzed, drug interactions, drug tolerance, postmortem interval, and the like.

INTRODUCTION

Forensic toxicology concerns the application of toxicology to situations that may have medicolegal review, and as a consequence, results must stand up to scrutiny in a court of law.[1] There are primarily three subdisciplines of forensic toxicology:

1. Postmortem toxicology, more recently referred to as death investigation toxicology.
2. Behavioral or human performance toxicology, which concerns
   a. Impaired driving as a result of alcohol and/or drugs consumption.
   b. Drug-facilitated sexual assault cases.
   c. Doping control. Screening of athletes for performance-enhancing substances is monitored by the World Anti-Doping Agency.[2] In this category must be included equine and canine toxicology testing, because entire laboratories are dedicated to this specific purpose.
3. Forensic workplace drug testing or drug urinalysis, which is performed as a preemployment and/or random monitoring of employees for illicit drugs or court-ordered testing of convicted drug offenders.

The author has nothing to disclose.
Toxicology Department, Cuyahoga County Region Forensic Science Laboratory, Cuyahoga County Medical Examiner's Office, 11001 Cedar Avenue, Cleveland, OH 44106, USA
E-mail address: jfwyman@cuyahogacounty.us

Clin Lab Med 32 (2012) 493–507
http://dx.doi.org/10.1016/j.cll.2012.06.005   labmed.theclinics.com
0272-2712/12/$ – see front matter Published by Elsevier Inc.

Closely related but in a category of its own is forensic drug chemistry.[3] This discipline is concerned with drug and chemical analysis, as is toxicology, but in regard to nonbiological specimens such as seized bales of marijuana, packets of synthetic cannabinoids, pills, "meth lab" reagent analyses, rocks of crack cocaine, and the like. Toxicology and drug chemistry laboratories often work together on different aspects of a case, especially when the laboratories are housed in the same facility. An important consideration when laboratories are in the same building is that extraction of drugs by each discipline must be accomplished in different rooms to avoid possible contamination of toxicology specimens by the relatively massive quantities of drug chemistry specimens.

To assist with the practice of forensic toxicology, a guide as to how the discipline should be performed is provided in the form of forensic toxicology laboratory guidelines, prepared by the Society of Forensic Toxicology (SOFT) and the Toxicology Section of the American Academy of Forensic Sciences (AAFS).[4] Also, at the time of this writing, a "draft" document entitled Scientific Working Group for Forensic Toxicology (SWGTOX) Standard Practices for Method Validation in Forensic Toxicology has been released for public comment. The practice of urine drug testing is defined by Mandatory Guidelines for Federal Workplace Drug Testing Programs, issued by the Department of Health and Human Services.[5] This review is restricted to the subdisciplines of postmortem and behavioral toxicology.

HOW FORENSIC TOXICOLOGY DIFFERS FROM CLINICAL TOXICOLOGY

Clinical toxicology is typically hospital-based, with the emergency room physicians being the primary customers. Analytical results must be obtained with speed to help confirm the therapeutic regimen for living patients, and an initial screen result by itself is sufficient for use in medical evaluation. Clinical analysts rarely are called about judicial matters, compared with forensic analysts. Quantification and confirmation of drug findings are not usually relevant to the treatment and often are not possible because of time constraints. Analytical instrumentation such as immunoassay provides fast but less specific results at a relatively lower cost. In larger laboratories with high-end analytical capability, physician-ordered therapeutic drug monitoring is performed.

By comparison, forensic toxicology can move at a slower and more comprehensive pace. Critical to the analytical process is a rigorous chain of custody from which the identity of the specimen is certain. Because the results for any case have the potential to end up in a court of law, there is a greater emphasis on specificity and accuracy in identifying potential toxicants. The cost of analysis is generally higher. For results to be reported, both a screen and confirmation must be performed using two different analytical procedures wherever possible; alternatively, when two analytical procedures are not available, a confirmation may be accomplished using (a) two different methods for extraction, (b) by demonstrating that a specific drug (metabolites) is present in two different specimens (eg, blood and urine), and/or (c) the drug is listed as part of the case history from the standpoint of medical record, prescription record, or death investigation.

CERTIFICATION AND ACCREDITATION

Forensic toxicology and all fields of forensic science are currently experiencing a period of accelerated change. The impetus for change came in 2009 with the National Academy of Sciences report[6] on the need for overhaul of forensic sciences in the United States. A major recommendation of this report was that forensic scientists should be certified in their specific discipline and laboratories should be accredited. Forensic toxicology certification is available primarily through two organizations: The American Board of Forensic Toxicology (ABFT)[7] and the Forensic Toxicology Certification Board.[8] Other certifications include the American Board of Clinical Chemistry, the American Board of Toxicology, the American Society for Clinical Pathology, and the National Registry of Certified Chemists. In addition to certification of analysts, certain states require that individuals performing toxicology testing on specimens from impaired drivers be licensed by the state's health departments.

Accreditation of toxicology laboratories can be accomplished through The ABFT and/or, based on the ISO 17025 Standards (Testing and Calibration Laboratories), through the American Society of Crime Laboratory Directors Laboratory Accreditation Board (ASCLD/LAB) program[9] or Forensic Quality Services, Inc.[10] Currently New York, Texas, and Oklahoma are the only states that require that toxicology laboratories be accredited. Other accrediting bodies include the National Laboratory Certification Program under the Substance Abuse and Mental Health Service Administration,[11] the National Association of Medical Examiners (NAME),[12] and the College of American Pathologists (CAP).[13]

TOXICOLOGY TESTING
Chain of Custody

In that the results of forensic toxicology testing may be used in court proceedings, the first necessary component of the testing process is to demonstrate the validity of test specimens. This demonstration is accomplished through the chain of custody,[14] which documents the chronologic disposition and condition of specimens from the time of collection to the time of disposal. The person initiating the chain of custody would typically provide the identity of the individual from whom the specimen was collected, what the specimen is, when it was collected (time and date) and by whom, including signatures. Tamper-evident tape with initials across the tape may be used to help maintain the integrity of the specimen. As the specimen moves through the transfer and testing process, printed names and signatures of releasing and receiving persons are recorded as are the time and date, the condition of the specimen, and the reason for transfer. Without correct, legible, and intact chain of custody documentation, the integrity and security of the specimens cannot be established, and the results of toxicology testing may be judged to be inadmissible to the court. The chain of custody form is often combined with the toxicology request form into a single document. The toxicology request form allows the selection of specific testing batteries such as a volatile screen, drug of abuse screen, comprehensive analysis, or other special testing requests.

Testing Service Provided

A standard testing battery within a forensic toxicology laboratory will include an alcohol (volatile) screen, a drug of abuse screen, electrolyte profile, and a comprehensive analysis. All screens include confirmation and quantitation of any positive results. Volatile analysis is most commonly performed by gas chromatography (GC), whereas drug of abuse screens are performed with immunoassay. Immunoassay is continually expanding to allow screening for tricyclic antidepressants, salicylate, acetaminophen, methadone, oxycodone, barbiturates, carisoprodol, promethazine, and other drugs. Some laboratories are transitioning to use of high-performance liquid chromatography (HPLC)/mass spectrometry (MS) for drug of abuse screens. Confirmations are most often performed by GC/MS analysis with or without derivatization of analytes or with HPLC/MS/MS, if this instrument is available. A comprehensive drug screen will include a volatile assay, an immunoassay of blood and urine, followed by GC/MS analysis of extracts of blood and urine. Electrolyte analysis is performed on vitreous humor rather than blood. Electrolyte values in blood are difficult to interpret after death, whereas sodium, chloride, magnesium, calcium, urea nitrogen, and creatinine remain essentially unchanged in the early postmortem period in the vitreous. Elevated glucose will persist in the vitreous allowing detection of hyperglycemia, whereas normal glucose levels fall and have no interpretive value. Other analytical procedures provided by laboratories fall into the category of "case-directed" testing. These are tests that are not routinely performed but are necessary based on the circumstances of the case. Examples include (1) carboxyhemoglobin assay in victims from house fires or decedents found in automobiles, (2) antipsychotic batteries for schizophrenics and manic/depressives, (3) anticonvulsant testing for seizure histories, (4) heavy metal assay for alleged poisonings, (5) gamma-hydroxybutyric acid in drug-facilitated sexual assault cases, and ethylene glycol as indicated. To complete case analysis, evaluation of evidence (patches, contaminated clothing, pill from gastric contents, drug paraphernalia (spoons, syringes, glass mirrors, wire mesh, and so forth) for drugs should be performed. If toxicology and drug chemistry are housed in the same laboratory area, evidence items can be analyzed by drug chemistry.

Matrices

The typical matrix for workplace or court-ordered drug testing is urine, although use of alternative matrices (sweat, hair, and/or saliva) are being examined to with increasing frequency.[15] Behavioral toxicology most frequently is performed on blood and/or urine specimens. Blood for forensic analysis is collected in gray top tubes containing the antimicrobial additive sodium fluoride and potassium oxalate as an anticoagulant. In that results may be presented in court, collection of blood in gray top tubes is an important forensic consideration. An often used defense strategy is to question the integrity of the specimen from the standpoint of in vitro *production* of ethanol. This argument is moot if the specimens are collected in gray top tubes and refrigerated. Interpretation of impairment from drug levels in urine is not possible, although some states have per se driving laws based on the concentration of drugs in urine. Whether the individual was under the influence of drugs or not cannot be established from urine results; all that can be reasonably known is that the individual was exposed to the drug.

Postmortem

Postmortem specimens are many and quite varied. If only an external examination is performed (no autopsy), then blood, urine, and vitreous humor are typically collected. During an autopsy, blood, urine, vitreous, bile, gastric, liver, spleen, kidney, brain, muscle, and hair may be collected. For fluids that have a finite volume such as gastric, bile, and urine, it is important to record the total volume present so that the total amount of drug can be calculated for the specific compartment. Other specimens that may be collected depending on the condition of the body and the toxicant of interest include nails, bone, meconium, cerebrospinal fluid, and blood clots. If the clot is connected to the cause of death, such as traumatic head injury with subdural hematoma, the clot should be homogenized and analyzed. This procedure will give some indication of blood constituents immediately following the time of the injury.

Hospital Specimens

Considerations for blood clots are similar for hospital specimens. If the decedent arrived at the hospital and admission specimens were collected, these are the most important specimens to analyze to obtain a valid interpretation of drug or alcohol contributions to the cause of death. Conversely, if admission specimens are not available and the hospital record reflects an extended hospital stay and/or transfusion/hemodilution, performing toxicology on postmortem specimens may be judged to be of little value. If family members indicate that they believe the hospital caused their loved one's death, then it is important that the laboratory analyze both admission blood (if available) and postmortem blood. Most hospitals keep collected specimens for a short time (eg, 1 week) before they are discarded. Blood banks may hold specimens for a longer period than the hospital. Death investigators are trained to act quickly to recover hospital specimens, if they are available. In some situations, hospitals may work with coroner/medical examiner offices to preserve blood when a medicolegal investigation is expected.

Other Analytical Issues for Consideration

1. **First assay.** The first test performed in a forensic analysis should be a screen for volatiles, in that ethanol, acetone, methanol, and other volatile constituents will be depleted in concentration each time the stopper is removed from the blood, vitreous, or urine tube.
2. **Dedicated instrumentation.** If the laboratory can afford the luxury of instruments dedicated to specific assays, this is an efficient way to operate. Time spent changing columns and loading new methods is avoided so that the flow of analytical assay is more productive.
3. **Drug stability.** Certain analytes (olanzapine, promethazine,[16] chlorpromazine, chlorprothixene, thioridazine, triflupromazine, ziprasidone,[17] zopiclone,[18] cyanide,[19] synthetic cathinones,[20] cocaine[21]) should be measured as soon as possible because of instability in storage. It is a good practice to characterize the stability of analytes as part of the validation of the analytical procedure. In most cases, stability is improved by refrigeration or freezing and by use of gray top tubes containing sodium fluoride.
4. **New drugs.** Laboratories must stay current with the constantly changing menu of available drugs, both prescribed and illicit. This ongoing task can be readily accomplished by attending annual meetings (SOFT, AAFS, The International Association of Forensic Toxicologists, NAME) and subscribing to relevant journals (*Journal of Analytical Toxicology* and the *Journal of Forensic Sciences*). SOFT's quarterly newsletter (*Tox Talk*) is an online publication containing a "New Drug" section.

   Additional requirements are

   a. To obtain new drug standards. Commercial drug companies include Cerilliant, Lipomed, Cayman Chemicals, and Grace Chemicals, to name a few. If a drug is not available it can sometimes be obtained by contacting the pharmaceutical company that manufactures the drug.
   b. GC/MS libraries must be updated continually. Commercial libraries appropriate for drug analysis including PMW (Pfleger, Maurer, Weber), NIST (National Institute of Standards and Technology), and Wiley Registry are available but expensive to acquire. Additional sources that are currently free are the RTI International "Forensic DB" (adopted from the AAFS library made available by Dr Graham Jones),[22] Scientific Working Group Drug library,[23] and of course, creating in-house libraries from acquired standards.

5. In GC and liquid chromatography (LC) analyses, to detect the possibility of carryover from one injection to the next, it is good practice to insert solvent blank

injections between control and case extracts. With autoinjectors, this process is easily accomplished using the instrument sequencing program.

PRINCIPLES OF QUALITY ASSURANCE

A quality assurance (QA) program is required to ensure that the laboratory produces consistently reliable drug/chemical identification and quantitation. Aspects of a QA program include

1. Competent analyst with access to continuing education. The number of analysts must be sufficient to handle the workload and provide testing services requested. If resources allow it, each analyst would ideally attend a national or international meeting each year. Certification in forensic toxicology should be encouraged. Subscription to relevant journals and acquisition of up-to-date toxicology texts are needed.
2. An adequate work environment with properly maintained instrumentation. Documentation of maintenance and corrective actions is required. A planned, systematic replacement of obsolete instruments should be incorporated into the laboratory budget.
3. Appropriate documentation of policies and procedures is required. This documentation is usually maintained as standard operating procedure manuals for administrative policies, quality assurance, analytical methods, accessioning of specimens (and disposal), training, safety, corrective actions, improvements, personnel training and competency, and the like.
4. Proficiency testing for volatile analytes and for drugs in blood, serum, and urine specimens is required. Typically, laboratories will subscribe to the CAP proficiency tests,[24] which will include series AL1 (American Association for Clinical Chemistry/CAP whole blood alcohol/ethylene glycol/volatiles, or AL2 (same but in serum), and forensic toxicology–criminalistics (FTC) and toxicology (T). These series require that the laboratory conduct proficiency testing three times each year for each series. For accreditation by the ABFT the AL1, FTC, and T series test must be performed.
5. Validation of new analytical methods prior to their use in case work may include the following criteria:
   a. Limit of detection (LOD), which is the lowest concentration detectable above background noise; usually three masses are used for confirmation.
   b. Limit of quantitation, which is normally the lowest concentration determined for the calibration curve.
   c. Linear range for an analyte is needed to establish the upper and lower concentrations at which the instrument response directly corresponds to the concentration of the drug/chemical. Determinations that exceed the linear range of the calibration curve must be repeated after the specimen has been appropriately diluted. Values that are less than the lowest concentration of the calibration curve, and greater than the LOD, are normally reported as less than that concentration or as "trace." Nonlinear relationships (eg quadratic) may exist for specific analytes, and use of instrument software to find the "best fit" curve will improve analytical accuracy.
   d. Accuracy is assessed through the use of controls. In order to validate the calibration curve, control concentrations must be analyzed. Preparation of controls should be from a source different from the source used to prepare the calibration curve, or else the curve will most assuredly be validated whether it is accurate or not. As much as is possible, calibrators and controls should be "matrix matched" (prepared in drug-free blood or urine). Depending on the assay, an acceptable accuracy may be as much as ± 20% from the target value. Volatile analysis of ethanol should not vary more than ± 5% of the

target value. Along with positive controls it is imperative that matrix-matched negative or blank controls be run with each assay. Calibration curves should be prepared with at least three different concentrations that define the linear range (low, middle, and high). Controls should be prepared at both high and low concentrations relative to the calibration curve, and both high and low controls should be included at the beginning and at the end of a batch analysis. A good practice is to include calibrations curve and control samples with each batch analysis, although some laboratories may make use of "historical" curves and freshly prepared controls.

e. Precision of the assay is measured as "within run" and "between run" and will involve determining the coefficient of variation (CV) for results from 10 to 20 separate assays. A CV of 10% or less is generally acceptable.

f. Specificity: interference from other analytes (those commonly identified in specific assays) should be determined by analyzing target analytes with and without other drugs present.

g. Recovery or extraction efficiency is determined by analyzing a known amount of analyte with and without extraction. The extraction efficiency will vary depending on the type and condition of the matrix. Decomposed specimens will severely decrease the analyst's ability to extract drugs from a matrix. Use of an appropriate internal standard should compensate for the variability in extraction efficiency. The best practice is to obtain deuterated homologs of specific analytes for use as internal standards. Laboratory resources may limit how many different deuterated internal standards can be used, because they are expensive to acquire.

h. Stability of analytes is often overlooked or not performed for need to place the assay in service. Knowing how long analytes will persist at the same concentration in a specific biological matrix is an important criterion that ideally, at some time, will be assessed.

i. Measure of uncertainty is a relatively new concept to forensic toxicology and is being progressively implemented in laboratories across the country. The need for determining uncertainty measurement for toxicology results was formally realized during a suppression hearing in Washington State.[25] Accreditation by the ASCLD/LAB-International Program[9] requires that uncertainty measures be known for specific analyses. Uncertainty measurement is how one determines the amount of variability that exists with a measured result, realizing that the true uncertainty can never be known. To determine what the uncertainty is requires identification of the most probable sources of uncertainty throughout the analytical process, followed by the formulation of an uncertainty budget. As an example, an uncertainty budget may be developed by considering the following:
- Reproducibility
- Purity of standards and reference materials
- Volumetric measurements as a function of maximum permissible errors and temperature
- Variability of calibrator solutions with temperature corrections
- Variability of pipette calibration
- Variability internal standard/sample delivery

Other uncertainties that are less significant than those listed previously may include
- Storage conditions
- Instrument effects
- Sample/matrix effects
- Computational effects.

The standard uncertainty is first calculated for each component of the budget. Different calculations must be applied to different types of uncertainty. Guides for these calculations are available.[26–30] Once standard uncertainties have been calculated, the combined uncertainty is calculated by squaring the value of each standard uncertainty, adding these together and then taking the square root of the sum of the squared uncertainties. When calculating the combined uncertainty, if the individual standard uncertainties for budget item is less than one-third of the maximum standard uncertainty, it can be ignored.

The final uncertainty determination is made by calculating the expanded uncertainty. This calculation requires a designated confidence interval of 95% or 99.7% (two or three standard deviations). The confidence interval is represented by 2 or 3, respectively, which is called the coverage factor "k." The expanded uncertainty is equal to the combined uncertainty multiplied by the coverage factor desired. The ASCLD/LAB-International Program is considering requiring that uncertainty measurement values be included on all toxicology reports, along with the measured value for the analyte.

An excellent reference for further reading on quality assurance is provided by Bramley and colleagues.[30]

POSTMORTEM INVESTIGATION

A strong forensic axiom is that no aspect of a death investigation is performed in isolation. There is communication with all staff members through a morning "viewing meeting" to discuss case history, medical records, pharmacy records, and the circumstances of the death. An important consideration is that "results of toxicology testing have to make sense" in light of the entire case findings. For example, GC/MS analysis of specimens and identification of cocaine with no detectable cocaine metabolites (benzoylecgonine, methyl ecgonine, cocaethylene) should give the toxicologist pause, in that cocaine does not present by itself in postmortem specimens. If this result occurs, the results of immunoassay screen for cocaine should be examined and a repeat analysis should be considered. Another example is a vitreous glucose greater than 600 mg/dL will often coincide with acetone in the blood and vitreous volatile analysis, because acetone is a product of diabetic ketoacidosis. An elevated glucose and acetone are complementary results. As is discussed later, heavy lungs following an overdose of central nervous system (CNS) depressants is an expected pathologic outcome.

Postmortem Interpretation of Toxicology Results

How does one determine that a drug concentration is therapeutic, toxic, or lethal? Unlike experimental toxicology, forensic toxicology must rely on case reports provided in the literature and on the experience of the toxicologist/pathologist. Many useful references are available to help guide the interpretation of postmortem drug levels.[31–36] An important aspect for interpreting toxicology results is knowledge of the specific case history, the medical record, and record of prescribed (or unprescribed) medications. Which forensic professional is responsible for drug interpretation will vary depending on the coroner or medical examiner office. The pathologist may rely on the toxicologist to provide the interpretation, or restrict the toxicologist to providing only the identity and concentration of drugs. The best practice is for the toxicologist and pathologist to have an open dialogue and collaborate on the interpretation of toxicology findings. In addition to the drug concentration in postmortem specimens, other factors to be considered are drug-drug interactions, the site of specimen collection, date of collection, the route of administration, and the length of time an individual has been taking a specific drug.

Signs of Toxic Pathology

Before toxicology testing begins, there may be evidence that a decedent was exposed to certain toxicants based on findings at the external exam or from gross or microscopic findings at autopsy. Examples include drugs in pockets of clothing, pill fragments in the mouth or nose, powder around the nostrils, and transdermal patches on the body or in the mouth. Examples of pathologic signs are a reddish hue to the skin produced by carbon monoxide; hemorrhagic gastritis, which could have been caused by heavy metals (arsenic or iron); cyanide, which also produces a rosy hue to the skin and may be detected by smell by approximately 20% to 40 % of the population at a threshold of .2 to 5 ppm[37]; Mees lines (white lines across the nail beds of fingers and toes), which may be produced by arsenic and thallium[38] along with a hyperkeratosis of the palms of the hands and soles of the feet; Burton's lines (blue or black lines along the margin of the gum and teeth)[39]; signs of allergic reactions such as a swollen tongue, rash, swollen airway, and voluminous lungs, which should prompt a request for test for β-tryptase levels and serum immunoglobulin E; and fresh needle punctures and/or old track marks of the skin, which suggest intravenous drug abuse.

Postmortem Redistribution

The propensity for certain drugs to have artifactually elevated concentrations in heart blood following death is known as postmortem redistribution (PMR).[40-42] Because the drug concentrations are not representative of blood levels when the individual was alive, use of drug concentrations in heart blood for interpretation can lead to erroneous conclusions about the cause of death. As the time interval between death and blood collection increases, the concentration of drug in heart blood increases. Blood collection sites farthest from the central compartment organs will be least affected by PMR. For purposes of interpretation, the preferential order of collection is femoral, then iliac, then subclavian vessels, and then heart. Drug levels in blood from the latter two collection sites are best left uninterpreted.

The phenomenon of PMR can be best characterized by thinking about drug distribution when a person is alive. Certain drugs are sequestered by central compartment organs (liver, lungs, and heart) at intracellular concentrations higher than the circulating blood. Examples of drugs that exhibit high levels of PMR are tricyclic antidepressants (eg, amitriptyline) and the analgesic propoxyphene. Ante-mortem concentrations of these drugs may be greater than tenfold higher in liver compared with circulating blood levels.[43] To maintain this concentration gradient during life requires energy and integrity of cell membranes. Cell death results in a loss of energy (oxidative phosphorylation of adenosine triphosphate ceases) and cell membranes are not maintained.

Determination of Dose in Postmortem Specimens is a Poor Practice

In clinical toxicology or therapeutic drug monitoring it is possible to calculate a dose consumed based on blood concentration, body weight, and the volume of distribution (V_d) of the drug as shown:

$$DOSE = Body\ Weight * Conc * V_d$$

In drug overdose cases it is natural to ask how many pills or capsules were consumed by the decedent. If prescription bottles are available, this number may be determined by counting the pills left in the bottle and correlating the pills consumed with how they were prescribed. To attempt to calculate dose after death based on postmortem blood concentration is a poor practice[44] for the following reasons:

1. V_d is never known for a specific individual and varies depending on body type (body mass index).
2. Whether a drug concentration is at steady state is not known (is distribution complete?).
3. PMR may elevate drug concentration from two- to tenfold.
4. V_d is based on plasma/serum concentrations, and postmortem toxicology is performed on whole blood.

The fallacy of calculating pill counts should be pointed out to any pathologist who has to respond to questions from family members and/or law enforcement. One should never present postmortem pill counts as evidence in court.

Cases of Suspected Overdose

Confirmation of suspected drug overdose cases should be accomplished using additional specimen analyses. If a lethal level of drug is determined for blood, then analysis of liver will demonstrate whether the high level is a systemic intoxication. Not following with a confirmation of systemic toxicity can sometimes lead to the wrong conclusions, such as when an implantable drug delivery system (drug pump) continues to release drug after death.

Tolerance or Loss of Tolerance

When evaluating drug levels in a deceased individual, it is important to review the history and/or medical records to determine the degree of tolerance, if any, that might have existed. Tolerance is an acquired phenomenon as a result of continued exposure to a chemical substance. Mechanisms of tolerance may include (a) an increase in metabolism of a drug as a result of metabolic enzyme induction and (b) desensitization of the receptor with a decrease in pharmacologic response. Individuals in a methadone maintenance program will have levels of methadone exceeding 1 mg/L,[31] whereas naïve users can expire from blood levels less than .2 mg/L. Whether tolerance to opiates, alcohol, or other drugs exists should be established before a drug level is ruled an overdose. Conversely, a loss of tolerance (opiates) by persons entering a drug rehabilitation program may result in their death if when they leave the program they resume their addiction at the same level as before they entered rehabilitation.

Conflicting Causes of Death in Litigated Cases

If the toxicologist's report provides an interpretation of the drug level detected (therapeutic, toxic, or lethal), it is always important to review the case history as to how the individual died. Even though a high level of heroin or cocaine might be considered lethal and a reasonable cause of death, reporting the drug as lethal could pose a problem if the immediate cause of death was a gunshot wound to the head and the case is a homicide. Reporting the drug level as lethal under these circumstances would provide the perpetrator a ready-made defense.

Specimen Collection in Decomposed Bodies

Depending on the state of decomposition, specimen collection from decomposed bodies can be quite limited. The traditional specimens of blood and vitreous are the first fluids to be lost; if the temperature is warm, these matrices may be gone after 48 hours decomposition. Other available specimens to be collected may include liver, kidney, muscle, bone, hair, nails, insect larvae, and/or soil beneath the remains. Liver, the traditional matrix used for interpretation of drug levels when blood is not available, should not be used for drug quantitation if the body is badly decomposed. After a few days decomposition, drug levels in liver can increase several-fold higher than what would have been measured at the time of death.[45] This change is a result of anatomic location (adjacent to the gastrointestinal tract) and fluid loss that decreases liver mass. This dramatic increase in liver drug concentration can easily lead to erroneous interpretation as to cause and manner of death. Drug concentration in muscle changes much less over time than that of liver and may be a more reliable matrix for interpretation.

Drug-Drug Interactions

Although there are many different categories of drug-drug interactions that one could describe (such as drugs and dietary supplements or drugs and food), the three principal interactions involve

1. **Induction and inhibition of metabolism.** Detoxification of drugs and chemicals in the body is carried out by reactions known as phase I and phase II metabolism. Phase I mostly involves oxidation and, to a lesser extent, reduction or hydrolysis of substrates, whereas phase II concerns the conjugation of substrates with small molecules such as glucuronide, glutathione, sulfate, glycine, acetate, and others.[46] Induction or inhibition of metabolism of one drug by another is almost always a result of phase I enzymes, principally hepatic cytochrome P-450 mixed function oxidases. A large body of drugs function as substrates, inducers, and/or inhibitors of this enzyme system.[47] One drug inducing the metabolism of another drug, by causing the production of more enzyme, may decrease the efficacy of the metabolized drug. Conversely, inhibition of cytochrome P-450 metabolism by a drug can cause an increase in toxicity of another drug. There are primarily five families of cytochrome P-450 found in humans.[48] Within these families, CYP3A4, CYP2D6, CYP2C9, CYP2C19, CYP1A2, and CYP2E1 are of importance.[46] Keeping track of which drugs serve as substrates, inducers, and/or inhibitors for which isozyme can be a daunting task. However, knowing that the vast majority ($\sim$ 75%) of drugs are metabolized by only two isozymes, CYP3A4 and CYP2D6,[46,49] helps to simplify; also that ethanol, in addition to alcohol dehydrogenase, is metabolized by CYP2E1. An in-depth discussion of cytochrome P-450 metabolism is outside the scope of this article. Suffice it to say that interpretation of postmortem toxicology results requires thinking about, and sometimes investigating the possibility of, induction or inhibition of metabolism of a drug by the presence of another drug. For the most part, however, drug-drug interaction as a result of induction or inhibition of metabolism is less of a concern with most drugs because the change in the drug concentration is typically small, and most drugs generally have a wide margin of safety and/or have multiple routes of metabolic elimination.
2. **Disruption of drug storage reservoirs.** The primary sites of drug storage are plasma proteins (albumin and acidic glycoproteins) and tissue (organs, muscle, and fat). If drugs bind to plasma proteins and/or tissues, they are no longer available to cause their pharmacologic effect. When another drug with a greater binding affinity for the binding site is introduced, the bound drug will become free to act. An example of toxicity as a result of drug-drug interaction is when ibuprofen is taken by a patient who is on warfarin. Use of ibuprofen (or other nonsteroidal

antiinflammatory drugs) with warfarin is contraindicated because ibuprofen will increase the concentration of warfarin and potentially cause unwanted hemorrhage.[50] Therefore, some appreciation for the propensity of a drug to displace another drug from plasma or tissue proteins can be gained by consulting the percent protein binding data.[31,36]

3. **Additive (synergistic) effects.** The most frequent type of drug-drug interaction that is encountered in postmortem, as well as human performance, toxicology is increased toxicity because of additive or synergistic effects. A pharmacologic effect common to numerous drug classes is CNS depression. CNS depression occurs as a direct or indirect result of consuming alcohol, opiates, barbiturates, benzodiazepines, tricyclic antidepressants, muscle relaxants, antihistamines, or lithium. Within these drug classes are as many as a hundred different drugs, so the likelihood of an individual consuming more than one CNS depressant is very possible. Individuals dying from depressant polypharmacy experience CNS depression, which leads to cardiac and respiratory depression (brain stem), followed by pulmonary edema (lung weight increases from a norm of 350 g to >1000 g) and death. Evidence of pulmonary edema may be visible at the death scene in the form of a "foam cone" on the nose and mouth. If a CNS depressant overdose is suspected as the cause of death, autopsy should reveal edematous lungs weighing in excess of 500 g along with a full bladder. Without these findings, a conclusion that the person died from an overdose of depressant drugs should be suspect.

Drug Polymorphisms and Pharmacogenetics (Pharmacogenomics)

Polymorphism means difference in phenotype between individuals, and pharmacogenetics is the study of the genetic variations that cause differences in the drug response among individuals.[46] These terms are used interchangeably, along with descriptions of "fast" and "slow" metabolizers. One of the first isozymes to be characterized was N-acetyltransferase 2, which causes the acetylation of isoniazid. Other drugs that have been shown to have variable metabolism as a result altered genetic makeup include succinylcholine (defects in pseudocholinesterase), nortriptyline and codeine (CYP2D6), mephenytoin (CYP2C19), warfarin, phenytoin, tolbutamide (CYP2C9*3), midazolam (CYP3A5), nicotine (CYP2A61B), methadone, selegiline, propofol, efavirenz, and cyclophosphamide (CYP2B6) .

SUMMARY

This article is intended to provide the reader an overview of principles, procedures, and practices in a modern forensic toxicology laboratory. Future trends in forensic toxicology may include a change in analytical procedures where LC tandem mass spectrometry, time of flight mass spectrometry, and/or capillary electrophoresis are the standard analytical methods. Certification of analyst and accreditation of laboratories will be a universal requirement. Laboratories will be able to minimize the use of paper by using electronic documentation. The overall effect of becoming a paperless laboratory will be an increase in efficiency, decrease in case turnaround times, and a reduction in cost. Interpretation of toxicology results from the perspective of pharmacogenetics will undoubtedly affect decisions concerning the cause and manner of death, as well as in legal proceedings. For further reading, an excellent introductory text, *Principles of Forensic Toxicology* has been provided by Levine.[51]

REFERENCES

1. The Forensic Toxicology Council. What is forensic toxicology? Published 2010. Available at: http://www.abft.org/files/WHAT%20IS%20FORENSIC%20TOXICOLOGY.pdf.   Accessed June 27, 2012.
2. United States Anti-Doping Agency. The World Anti-Doping Agency (WADA) prohibited list. Available at: http://www.usada.org/prohibited-list/?gclid=CPaOIYiaqq8CFYEQ NAodEHcDZQ. Accessed June 27, 2012.
3. Siegel JA. Forensic identification of illicit drugs. In: Saferstein R, editor. Forensic science handbook, vol. II. Upper Saddle River (NJ): Pearson/Prentice Hall; 2005. p. 111–74.
4. Society of Forensic Toxicologists/American Academy of Forensic Sciences. SOFT/AAFS forensic laboratory guidelines. 2006 version. Available at: http://www.soft-tox.org/files/Guidelines_2006_Final.pdf. Accessed June 27, 2012.
5. Department of Health and Human Services, Substance Abuse and Mental Health Services Administration. Mandatory guidelines for federal workplace drug testing programs. Federal Register 2008;73(228). Available at: http://www.gpo.gov/fdsys/pkg/FR-2008-11-25/pdf/E8-26726.pdf. Accessed June 27, 2012.
6. Committee on Identifying the Needs of the Forensic Sciences Community, National Research Council. Strengthening forensic science in the United States: a path forward. Washington (DC): The National Academies Press; 2008.
7. The American Board of Forensic Toxicology home page. Available at: http://www.abft.org/. Accessed June 27, 2012.
8. The Forensic Toxicology Certification Board home page. Available at: http://home.usit.net/~robsears/ftcb/index.htm. Accessed June 27, 2012.
9. American Society of Crime Laboratory Directors/Laboratory Accreditation Board. Programs of accreditation. Available at: http://www.ascld-lab.org/programs/prgrams_of_accreditation_index.html. Accessed June 27, 2012.
10. Forensic Quality Services home page. Available at: http://www.forquality.org/. Accessed June 27, 2012.
11. Substance Abuse and Mental Health Services Administration home page. Available at: http://www.samhsa.gov/. Accessed June 27, 2012.
12. National Association of Medical Examiners home page. Available at: http://thename.org/index.php. Accessed June 27, 2012.
13. College of American Pathologists home page. Available at: http://www.cap.org. Accessed June 27, 2012.
14. Houck M, Siegel JA. Fundamentals of forensic science. San Diego (CA): Elsevier Academic Press; 2006. p. 631.
15. Jenkins, AJ, editor. Drug testing in alternate biological specimens. Totowa (NJ): I lumana Press; 2010.
16. Karinen, R, Oiestad, EL, Andresen, W, et al. Comparison of the stability of stock solutions of drugs of abuse and other drugs stored in a freezer, refrigerator, and at ambient temperature for up to one year. J Anal Toxicol 2011;35(8):583–90.
17. Saar, E, Gerostamolulos, D, Drummer, OH, et al. Assessment of the stability of 30 antipsychotic drugs in stored blood specimens. Forensic Sci Int 2012;215(1–3): 152–8.
18. Jantos, R, Vermeeren, A, Sabljic, D, et al. Degradation of zopiclone during storage of spiked and authentic whole blood and matching dried blood spots. Int J Legal Med 2012. [Epub ahead of print].
19. Rodkey FL, Robertson RF. Analytical precautions in measurement of blood cyanide. Clin Chem 1978;24(12):2184–5.

20. Sorensen LK. Stability of cathinones in whole blood samples [P090]. Presented at the Joint Meeting of the Society of Forensic Toxicologists and The International Association of Forensic Toxicologists. San Francisco, September 25–30, 2011.

21. Giorgi SN, Meeker JE. A 5-year study of common illicit drugs in blood. J Anal Toxicol 1995;19(6):392–8.

22. RTI International. RTI International launches new spectral database for forensic laboratory, research, law enforcement [news release]. Available at: http://www.rti.org/news.cfm?nav=6&objectid=BC4CE78F-5056-B100-315CE42685250E90. Accessed June 27, 2012.

23. Scientific Working Group for the Analysis of Seized Drugs. SWGDRUG mass spectral library. Available at: http://www.swgdrug.org/ms.htm. Accessed June 27, 2012.

24. College of American Pathologists. Reference resources and publications. Available at: http://www.cap.org/apps/cap.portal?_nfpb=true&_pageLabel=reference. Accessed June 27, 2012.

25. Snohomish County District Court, Cascade Division, State of Washington v. Weimer, George G., #7036A-09D, memorandum decision on motion to suppress. Available at: http://www.cacj.org/documents/SF_Crime_Lab/Case_Law/WA-State-Decision-analysis-of-error-rate-is-applicable-across-many-fields-of-forensic-science-especially-drug-testing.pdf. Accessed June 27, 2012.

26. LeBeau AM. The tools for DIY methods validation, "Uncertainty in Forensic Toxicology". Presented at the Society of Forensic Toxicologists Workshop. Richmond (VA), October 18, 2010.

27. Meyer VR. Measurement uncertainty. J Chromatog A 2007;1158:15–24.

28. Ellison SL, Rosslein M, Wiliams A, editors. EURACHEM/CITAC Guide. Quantifying uncertainty in analytical measurement. 2nd edition. 2000. Available at: http://www.measurementuncertainty.org/pdf/QUAM2000-1.pdf. Accessed June 27, 2012.

29. Adams TM. G104 - A2LA. Guide for estimation of measurement uncertainty in testing. Published 2002. Available at: http://www.a2la.org/guidance/est_mu_testing.pdf. Accessed June 27, 2012.

30. Bramley RK, Bullock DG, Garcia JR. Quality control and assessment. In Jickells S, Negrusz A, editors. Clarke's analytical forensic toxicology. London (Chicago): Pharmaceutical Press; 2008.

31. Baselt RC, editor. Disposition of toxic drugs and chemicals in man. 9th edition. Seal Beach (CA): Biomedical Publications; 2009.

32. Molina DK. Handbook of forensic toxicology for medical examiners. Boca Raton (FL): CRC Press; 2010.

33. Winek CL, Wahba WW, Winek CL Jr. Winek's drug & chemical blood-level data 2001. Available at: http://medschool.slu.edu/abmdi/uploads/files/Winek%20tox%20data%202001.pdf. Accessed June 27, 2012.

34. Meyer FP. Indicative therapeutic and toxic drug concentrations in plasma: a tabulation. Int J Clin Pharmacol Ther 1994;32(2):71–81.

35. Office of the Chief Medical Examiner, Chapel Hill, NC. Toxic drug concentrations. Published 2009. Available at: http://www.ocme.unc.edu/toxicology/OCME_Tox.html. Accessed June 27, 2012.

36. Moffat AC, Osselton MD, Widdop B, editors. Clarke's analysis of drugs and poisons, vol. 2. 3rd edition. London: Pharmaceutical Press; 2004.

37. Ellenhorn MJ. Ellenhorn's medical toxicology: diagnosis and treatment of human poisoning. 2nd edition. Baltimore; Philadelphia: Williams and Wilkins, A Waverly Company; 1997. p. 1477.

38. Chauhan S, D'Cruz S, Singh R, et al. Mees' lines. Lancet 2008;372(9647):1410. Available at: http://www.thelancet.com/journals/lancet/article/PIIS0140-6736(08) 61587-1/fulltext. Accessed June 27, 2012.

39. Nogue S, Culla A. Images in clinical medicine. Burton's line. N Engl J Med 2006;354: e21. Available at: http://www.nejm.org/doi/full/10.1056/NEJMicm050064. Accessed June 27, 2012.

40. Anderson WH, Prouty RW. Postmortem redistribution of drugs. In: Baselt RC, editor. Advances in analytical toxicology, vol 2. Foster City (CA): Biomedical Publications; 1989. p. 70–102.

41. Pounder DJ, Jones GR. Post-mortem drug redistribution—a toxicological nightmare. Forensic Sci Int 1990;45(3):253–63.

42. Drummer OH, Gerostamoulos J. Postmortem drug analysis: analytical and toxicological aspects. Ther Drug Monit 2002;24(2):199–209.

43. Baselt RC, editor. Disposition of toxic drugs and chemicals in man. 8th edition. Seal Beach (CA): Biomedical Publications. 2008. p. 51, 1332.

44. Jones G. SOFT position statement on the use of volume of distribution calculations for drugs in postmortem cases. ToxTalk 2005;29(2):9.

45. Wyman JF, Dean DE, Yinger R, et al. The temporal fate of drugs in decomposing porcine tissue. J Forensic Sci 2011;56(3):694–9.

46. Correia MA. Drug biotransformation, In: Katzung BG, Masters SB, Trevor, AJ, editors. Basic and clinical pharmacology. 11th edition. San Francisco: McGraw Hill Lange; 2009. p. 53–66.

47. Indiana University School of Medicine, Department of Medicine, Division of Clinical Pharmacology. P-450 drug interaction table. Available at: http://medicine.iupui.edu/clinpharm/ddis/table.aspx. Accessed June 27, 2012.

48. The Human Cytochrome P450 (CYP) Allele Nomenclature Committee. The human cytochrome P450 (CYP) allele nomenclature database. Available at: http://www.cypalleles.ki.se. Accessed June 27, 2012.

49. Veith H, Southall N, Huang R, et al. Comprehensive characterization of cytochrome P450 isozyme selectivity across chemical libraries. Nat Biotechnol 2009;27:1050–5.

50. Prybys KM. Deadly drug interactions in emergency medicine. Emerg Med Clin North Am 2004;22(4):845–65.

51. Levine B. Principles of forensic toxicology. 3rd edition. Washington, DC: AACC Press; 2009.

Pharmacogenomics and the Future of Toxicology Testing

Yash Pal Agrawal, MBBS, PhD*, Hanna Rennert, PhD

KEY WORDS

- Toxicology • Pharmacogenomics • Pharmacogenetics • Autopsy • Drugs

KEY POINTS

- Pharmacogenomics is a useful tool in clinical toxicology for the characterization of many gene polymorphisms associated with different pharmacokinetics or pharmacodynamics of exogenously administered drugs.
- These genetic variants may determine ranges of variation in such fundamental aspects as drug-metabolizing enzymes, drug transporters, drug receptors, or targets of drug action.
- Toxicologically significant drugs for which the FDA has required the manufacturer to identify relevant pharmacogenomics markers on the label include carisoprodol, citalopram, codeine, and risperidone.
- *CYP2D6* variant alleles can result in four metabolic phenotypes—ultrarapid metabolizers, extensive metabolizers, intermediate metabolizers, and poor metabolizers—that demonstrate significant differences in opiate metabolism.
- For personalized medicine, combining pharmacogenomics testing with therapeutic drug monitoring may allow the identification of individuals who need lower or higher doses, or even a different drug.

INTRODUCTION

The human genome consists of about 30,000 genes comprised of billions of nucleotides. Although the DNA of any two different persons is 99% identical, variant sequences can and do occur in individuals. Variants that are found in more than 1% of the population are called polymorphisms, of which the most common type is the single nucleotide polymorphism (SNP). Deletion, insertion, and tandem repeats are other types of polymorphisms collectively termed copy number variations (CNVs). The role of inheritance in individual variation to drug response has been studied extensively; when applied to specific genes it has been called pharmacogenetics (PGt), and when applied to the whole genome it has been referred to as pharmacogenomics

The authors have nothing to disclose.
Department of Pathology and Laboratory Medicine, Weill Cornell Medical College, 525 East 68th Street, New York, NY 10065, USA
* Corresponding author.
E-mail address: yaa2004@med.cornell.edu

Clin Lab Med 32 (2012) 509–523
http://dx.doi.org/10.1016/j.cll.2012.07.009
0272-2712/12/$ – see front matter © 2012 Elsevier Inc. All rights reserved.

labmed.theclinics.com

Table 1
Selected drugs of toxicological significance with pharmacogenomic biomarkers listed on FDA drug label

Drug	Biomarker	Therapeutic Area	Significance
Carisoprodol	CYP2C19	Musculoskeletal pain	Reduced CYP2C19 activity; reduced metabolism of carisoprodol, and increased risk of drug toxicity
Atomoxetine	CYP2D6	Psychiatry	Initiate therapy with low dose in CYP2D6 poor metabolizers
Aripiprazole	CYP2D6 CYP3A4	Psychiatry	Reduced dose in poor metabolizers of CYP2D6 or patients on CYP3A4 inhibitors
Clobazam	CYP2C19	Neurology	Dose reduction in poor metabolizers of CYP2C19
Citalopram	CYP2C19	Psychiatry	Dose restriction in poor metabolizers of CYP2C19
Codeine	CYP2D6	Analgesia	Impact on dose in ultra- and poor metabolizers of CYP2D6
Flurbiprofen	CYP2C9	Rheumatology	Reduced dose in poor metabolizers of CYP2C9
Iloperidone	CYP2D6 CYP3A4	Psychiatry	Reduced dose in patients on CYP2D6 and CYP3A4 inhibitors
Risperidone	CYP2D6 CYP3A4	Psychiatry	Dose modulation needed in patients on CYP2D6 inhibitors (eg, fluoxetine) and CYP3A4 inducers (eg, carbamazepine, phenytoin, phenobarbital)

(PGx). For the purposes of this review, the terms PGx and PGt are used interchangeably.[1] Many excellent reviews have been published on various aspects of PGx. Implementation of PGx from a laboratory perspective,[2] various clinical interpretation guidelines,[3–6] as well as PGx as applied to clinical therapeutics in various specialties of medicine has been discussed.[7–9] Most of these reviews cover the therapeutic use of a pharmacologic drug/marker combination. However, occasionally the body's response to the drug is toxicity, possibly caused by an adverse drug reaction due to the interindividual variations in drug response.

There are many polymorphisms in several of the human genes associated with pharmacokinetics or pharmacodynamics of exogenously administered drugs. These variants typically characterize drug-metabolizing enzymes, drug transporters, drug receptors, or targets of drug action.[10] Currently the U.S. Food and Drug Administration (FDA) lists[11] more than 100 drugs that have a reference to a pharmacogenetic biomarker in a drug label. Examples from these drugs that may be seen in a toxicology practice are listed in **Table 1**.

In a toxicology setting, one may find patients who experience drug toxicity or drug adverse reactions at drug doses that are therapeutic to the vast majority of the population. Multiple factors are involved in such individual variations to drug response, including genetic, environmental (eg smoking and alcohol consumption), and physiologic (age, sex) factors as well as drug–drug interactions. The genetic factors can be broadly grouped into polymorphisms of proteins involved in drug targeting (ie, pharmacodynamics) and polymorphisms of proteins and enzymes related to drug transport (eg, P-glycoprotein, ABCB1) and metabolism (pharmacokinetics).[10]

GENETIC POLYMORPHISMS OF DRUG TARGETS

In general, with respect to the practice of clinical toxicology, individual variation in drug response due to polymorphism of drug targets is an infrequent cause of toxicity.

Thus, for example, polymorphism of the *ADRB2* gene,[10] which encodes the target receptor of β-agonists such as albuterol, has been described. These polymorphisms can result in a stronger and more rapid response to albuterol compared to the normal albuterol gene sequence. Another classic example relates to the inhibitory effect of warfarin on *VKORC1* (Vitamin K Epoxide Reductase Complex subunit 1 complex. *VKORC1* is involved in reduced production of vitamin K, which is necessary for γ-carboxylation of coagulation proteins. Warfarin therapy thus inhibits the production of normal coagulation proteins and causes an anticoagulant effect. Polymorphisms in *VKORC1* can cause resistance to warfarin treatment.[7] More commonly, drug toxicity is due to induction or inhibition of enzymes responsible for drug metabolism or transport of the drug in question.

GENETIC POLYMORPHISMS OF DRUG-METABOLIZING ENZYMES

Polymorphisms in liver cytochrome P450 group of enzymes which mediate Phase I and Phase II metabolism of drugs are very important with respect to an individual's susceptibility to toxicity or drug adverse reaction.[12] Phase I reactions (drug modification reactions) lead to functionalization of the drug by addition or uncovering of functional groups (eg, oxidation or hydrolysis) that can undergo subsequent metabolism by phase II enzymes. Phase II reactions are biosynthetic in nature (drug conjugation reactions), for example, glucuronidation or sulfation of drugs (eg, morphine is glucuronidated via UGT2B7). Many of the drug compounds are lipophilic in nature, and phase II reactions help the metabolites become water soluble, which can then be more easily excreted by the kidneys. Induction or inhibition of the liver CYP450 enzymes can increase or decrease drug metabolism with possible drug toxicity or failure of therapeutic effect. Hundreds of CYP enzymes have been described that are involved in the metabolism of drugs. For the most part, these enzymes do not have a major significance from a toxicological aspect and are not evaluated in routine clinical practice.[3,13] Allelic variation in noncytochrome P450 enzymes can also be important, for example, *UGT1A1* for irinotecan metabolism and glucuronidation of drugs. Of the CYP enzymes,[14] it is estimated, that, for example, CYP2D6 alone is responsible for metabolism of about 25% of drugs in clinical use.

Drug toxicity as well as drug abuse can result in emergency department (ED) visits. No doubt, some of these visits are the result of unexpected toxic effects due to individual variation in drug response, although exact data are difficult to come by. An estimate of the extent of the problem, as well as the key drug categories that may be important from a pharmacogenomic toxicology aspect in ED visits in the United States, can be gleaned from the Substance Abuse and Mental Health Services Administration (SAMHSA) data.[15] The U.S. Drug Abuse Warning Network (DAWN) estimates that in 2009 there were 2.1 million ED visits related to drug misuse or abuse. The most commonly abused pharmaceutical drug categories are listed in **Table 2**.

Further breakdown of the toxicologically significant pharmaceutical drugs and illicit drugs are indicated in **Tables 3** and **4** respectively. This review discusses the role of PGx to evaluate possible toxicity from some of the central nervous system (CNS) agents and illicit drugs that are commonly misused. We focus on CYP2D6 as the pharmacogenomic marker because it has considerable clinical relevance in toxicology. We also use CYP2D6 to introduce several of the primary pharmacogenomic databases available on the Web and then finally discuss some of the future technologies that may be relevant for PGx testing.

Table 2
Distribution of 2.1 million ED visits for drug misuse (2009)

Reason	%
Pharmaceutical drugs	35.3
Illicit drugs	23
Illicit drugs + alcohol	10.2
Pharmaceuticals + alcohol	11
Pharmaceuticals + Illicit drugs	10
Alcohol (aged 20 or younger)	6.7
Pharmaceuticals + illicit drugs + alcohol	3.9

Data from Substance Abuse and Mental Health Services Administration, Drug Abuse Warning Network, 2009: National estimates of drug-related emergency department visits. HHS Publication No. (SMA) 11-4659, DAWN Series D-35. Rockville (MD): Substance Abuse and Mental Health Services Administration, 2011. Available at: http://www.samhsa.gov/data/2k11/DAWN/2k9DAWNED/HTML/DAWN2k9ED.htm. Accessed August 8, 2012.

PHARMACOGENOMICS OF OPIATES

As shown in **Tables 3** and **4**, CNS narcotic pain relievers are abused frequently and account for a large number of ED visits. These commonly include the opium poppy (*Papaver somniferum*) derived alkaloid drugs, morphine, codeine, and heroin. Morphine is prepared from opium; codeine and heroin are obtained via chemical modification of morphine. Codeine is obtained by formation of methylmorphine and heroin by diacetylation of morphine. Hydromorphone, oxymorphone, hydrocodone, and oxycodone can be made via chemical modifications of morphine in vivo or by chemical synthesis. When evaluating opiate toxicity, it is necessary to be aware of the metabolites as well as interconversion of one drug to another. The clinical toxicology of the opiates, sample collection, and metabolites have been discussed recently.[16,17]

Table 3
The most commonly abused pharmaceutical drug groups responsible for ED visits, 2009

Pharmaceutical Drug	% of ED Visits	ED Visits
Psychotherapeutic agents • Antidepressants • Antipsychotics	12.3	132,482
CNS agents[a]	73.3	791,385
Respiratory agents	3.3	35,867
Cardiovascular agents	4.3	46,416
Gastrointestinal agents, hormones, metabolic agents, nutritional products	6	63,876

For details, see Substance Abuse and Mental Health Services Administration, Drug Abuse Warning Network, 2009: National estimates of drug-related emergency department visits. HHS Publication No. (SMA) 11-4659, DAWN Series D-35. Rockville (MD): Substance Abuse and Mental Health Services Administration, 2011. Available at: http://www.samhsa.gov/data/2k11/DAWN/2k9DAWNED/HTML/DAWN2k9ED.htm. Accessed August 8, 2012.
[a] The most common CNS agents were the narcotic pain relievers (oxycodone, hydrocodone, methadone), as well as non-narcotic pain relievers (acetaminophen, ibuprofen, naproxen). Sedatives such as benzodiazepines along with alprazolam were commonly misused.

Table 4
The most commonly abused illicit drugs singly or in combination in ED visits, 2009

Drug	%	Number of ED Visits
Cocaine	43.4	422,896
Marijuana	38.7	376,467
Alcohol	29.9	291,553
Heroin	21.9	213,118
Stimulants (eg, amphetamine, methamphetamine)	9.6	93,562
Others (eg, phencyclidine [PCP], methylenedioxymethylamphetamine [MDMA], hallucinogens, lysergic acid diethylamide [LSD], γ-hydroxybutyric acid [GHB], ketamine, inhalants)	<4	<39,000

The % totals do not add up to 100 because some drugs were taken in combination with other illicit drugs.
Data from Substance Abuse and Mental Health Services Administration, Drug Abuse Warning Network, 2009: National estimates of drug-related emergency department visits. HHS Publication No. (SMA) 11-4659, DAWN Series D-35. Rockville (MD): Substance Abuse and Mental Health Services Administration, 2011. Available at: http://www.samhsa.gov/data/2k11/DAWN/2k9DAWNED/HTML/DAWN2k9ED.htm. Accessed August 8, 2012.

Codeine

As seen in **Fig. 1**, Codeine is a prodrug that is converted to the active morphine[18] via CYP2D6. Even though the formation of morphine is a minor pathway (approximately 10% of dose), there is serious risk of toxicity in the ultra-rapid metabolizers, see **Table 5**. About 80% of the codeine dose is converted to inactive codeine-6-glucuronide. Norcodeine does not have analgesic activity.

The various active and inactive metabolites of opioid compounds have been described.[17] The role of CYP2D6 genotyping in patients taking codeine is to identify both the ultrarapid metabolizers (risk of systemic toxicity) as well as the poor metabolizers (risk of inadequate relief of pain). Comprehensive Clinical Pharmacogenetics Implementation (CPIC) guidelines for codeine therapy in the context of CYP2D6 genotype have been published.[18] These discuss in detail the challenges of CYP2D6 genotyping, techniques, reference laboratories, and allele frequencies in major ethnic groups as well as the common polymorphisms that are seen in clinical practice.

Polymorphisms of CYP2D6 can result in four metabolic phenotypes: ultrarapid, extensive, intermediate, and poor metabolizers (**Table 5**).

Common CYP2D6 Molecular Assay Platforms

Several commercial as well as laboratory-developed tests (LDTs) are now available for pharmacogenetic testing; three of the common ones are discussed briefly. The **Roche Amplichip P450** FDA-cleared Kit (Roche Diagnostics, Indianapolis, IN, USA), which simultaneously analyzes a patient's genotype for CYP2D6 and CYP2C19, was one of the first steps toward addressing adverse drug reactions (ADRs) and the introduction of pharmacogenetic testing into the clinical environment. This assay tests for 27 alleles, including 7 duplications in the CYP2D6 gene in a single reaction. In this assay genomic DNA is amplified in two multiplex polymerase chain reaction (PCR) reactions. After fragmentation and labeling, the PCR products are denatured and hybridized to a microarray. The signal is then detected on an Affymetrix GeneChip

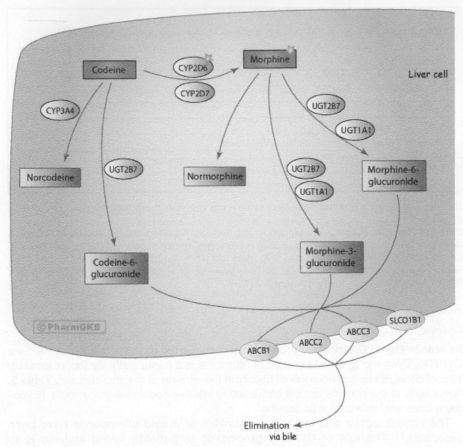

Elimination
via bile

Fig. 1. Candidate genes involved in codeine and morphine metabolism. (Figure ©PharmGKB and Stanford University; reprinted with permission.)

Scanner 3000Dx (Affymetrix, Santa Clara, CA, USA) and alleles assigned automatically by AmpliChip CYP450_US Data Analysis Software that classifies individuals into four principal CYP2D6 phenotypes: ultrarapid, extensive, intermediate, and poor metabolizers.

The **Luminex xTag 2D6 Mutation Detection Kit** (Luminex Molecular Diagnostics, Austin, TX, USA) simultaneously screens for 15 variants. In this assay, genomic DNA is amplified in two PCR reactions, and alleles are discriminated using allele-specific primer extension (ASPE) and hybridization to a universal microsphere array. Genotypes are detected on a Luminex 100 IS System and assigned using the proprietary TDAS software.

The **AutoGenomics INFINITI 2D6 Mutation Detection Kit** (AutoGenomics, Inc., Carlsbad, CA, USA) simultaneously screens for 15 variants. After PCR, alleles are distinguished using ASPE, resulting in incorporation of fluorescent CY5-dCTP. Extended primers are then hybridized to complementary capture probes immobilized on the BioFilmChip, and fluorescence is quantitated after scanning of the microarray using an integrated optics unit. Genotypes were assigned automatically by the proprietary software.

Table 5
Pharmacogenomic aspects of CYP2D6 metabolism of codeine

Phenotype	Example of Diplotype	Clinical Significance	% of Population	Clinical Application
Ultrarapid metabolizers	*1/*1 XN, *2/*2XN	Because more than two copies of functional alleles are present, there is increased conversion of codeine to morphine. This increases risk of toxicity.	1–2	A baby died of morphine poisoning after breast feeding by a mother (ultrarapid metabolizer) who was prescribed codeine[33]
Extensive metabolizer	Two full function/ reduced function alleles, or one full function allele in combination with reduced function/ nonfunctional allele *1/*1, *1/*2, *2/*2, *1/*41, *1/ *4, *2/*5, *10/*10	Normal codeine metabolism,	77–92	
Intermediate metabolizer	One reduced activity allele or a defective allele *4/*10, *5/*41	Reduced formation of morphine; drug may be less effective at usual doses.	2–11	
Poor metabolizer	No functional alleles, *4/*4, *4/*5, *5/*5, *4/*6	Very little morphine is formed; drug may be ineffective.	5–10	

Data from Crews KR, Gaedigk A, Dunnenberger HM, et al and Clinical Pharmacogenetics Implementation Consortium. Clinical Pharmacogenetics Implementation Consortium (CPIC) guidelines for codeine therapy in the context of cytochrome P450 2D6 (CYP2D6) genotype. Clin Pharmacol Ther 2012;91:321–6.

PHARMACOGENOMICS OF SYNTHETIC AND SEMISYNTHETIC OPIATES
Heroin

Heroin undergoes significant inactivation by first-pass metabolism in the liver, so it is not consumed orally. It is converted by hCE1 and hCE2 to the active 6-monoacetylmorphine (6-MAM), which is further converted to morphine.[19,20] The presence of 6-MAM in urine differentiates heroin use from morphine. Heroin and 6-MAM are more lipid soluble than morphine, and thus enter the brain and cause toxicity. There is no definite advantage to pharmacogenomic testing in relation to heroin toxicity.

Morphine

Morphine is glucuronidated to the active morphine-6-glucuronide by UGT2B7 and UGT1A1, as well as the inactive compounds morphine-3-glucuronide and normorphine

Table 6
Opioid metabolites that can be confused with exogenously consumed drugs of abuse

Opioid	Inactive Metabolites	Active Metabolites	Active Metabolites That Mimic Abused Drugs
Morphine	Normorphine	Morphone-3-glucuronide morphone-6-glucuronide	Hydromorphone
Hydromorphone	Minor metabolites	Hydromorphone-3 glucuronide	None
Hydrocodone	Norhydrocodone	None	Hydromorphone
Codeine	Norcodeine	None	Hydrocodone Morphine
Oxycodone	None	Noroxycodone	Oxymorphone
Oxymorphone	Oxymorphone-3-glucuronide	6-Hydroxy-oxymorphone	None
Tramadol	Nortramadol	O-desmethyltramadol	None
Heroin	Normorphine	6-Monoacetylmorphine	Morphine

Data from Smith HS. Opioid metabolism. Mayo Clin Proc 2009;7:613–24; with permission. Copyright Elsevier.

(**Fig. 1**). In postmortem samples, hydrolysis of glucuronidated morphine metabolites back to morphine can complicate interpretation of test results. Acute ingestion of morphine could be suspected in the presence of morphine in blood but not in urine. Polymorphisms of UGTB7 and UGT1A1 do not seem to have any significant effects related to morphine clearance or AUC profiles.[19,20]

Tramadol

A synthetic opioid, tramadol is converted to its active metabolite O-demethytramadol by CP2D6 and excreted in urine. The active metabolite is two to four times more potent than the parent drug. The N-demethylation pathway is less well characterized. Similar to its actions in codeine metabolism, CYP2D6 plays an important role. The ratios of tramadol to O-demethytramadol were measured in postmortem specimens and showed a clear decrease in their ratio as the number of functional alleles increased.[19,21] Poor metabolizers showed a high nonresponse rate to tramadol, and thus poor efficacy of tramadol analgesia.

Other Semisynthetic and Synthetic Opioids

The opioids hydrocodone and oxycodone are O-demethylated by CYP2D6 to hydromorphone and oxymorphone, respectively. It is not clear if the ultrarapid metabolizer status of CYP2D6 has any clear significance with respect to hydrocodone and oxycodone. Oxycodone, hydrocodone are not important compounds from a clinical pharmacogenomic testing aspect, except that the endogenously produced metabolites can sometimes be difficult to distinguish from exogenously consumed drugs of abuse (**Table 6**). The pharmacogenomics of these and other synthetic opiates such as methadone, fentanyl, and buprenorphine have been reviewed elsewhere.[19]

PHARMACOGENOMICS IN PAIN MANAGEMENT

When physicians use pain management drugs, their aim is to personalize the pain management regimen to the patient. Pharmacogenomics testing along with therapeutic drug monitoring in poor metabolizers or ultrametabolizers of drugs may allow one to identify those individuals who need a lower dose, a higher dose, or even a different drug. Apart from the role of *CYP2D6* in opiate metabolism discussed in the preceding text, other polymorphic genes such as *ABCB1, CYP3A4* have not gained wide clinical usage.[22]

PHARMACOGENOMICS OF ALCOHOL INGESTION

Alcohol alone or in combination with illicit/pharmaceutical drugs accounts for more than 25% of ED visits annually (**Table 2**). An individual's response to alcohol ingestion is dependent on many factors, including age, sex, body weight, and amount of ethanol ingested. Identical doses of ethanol may produce very different adverse effects in different individuals. Routine pharmacogenomic testing does not currently allow one to differentiate between an individual's response to alcohol or even recovery from insobriety. This is because multiple genes have been implicated in alcohol metabolism, including genes for alcohol dehydrogenase (*ALDH*), *CYP2E1*, µ-opioid receptor gene (*OPRM1*), γ-aminobutyric acid (GABA) receptor, serotonin transporter (rh5-HTTLPR), and acetylcholine receptor alpha 3 (CHRNA3). At the present time, there is no widely accepted pharmacogenomic test available for use in cases of alcohol-related toxicity.[23]

PHARMACOGENOMICS AND AUTOPSY EXAMINATION

The preferred sample type is whole blood. This has the advantage that the same sample can be used for toxicological drug/metabolite examination, as well as for pharmacogenomic testing. The preanalytical factors,[24] drug metabolite stability, and tissue redistribution of toxicologically relevant drugs have been discussed.[25-27] Some postmortem studies that utilized pharmacogenomics are described in **Table 7**. The role of pharmacogenomic testing in DUID (driving under the influence of drugs) cases is to determine if the person was impaired (abusing the drug) or is taking a drug as prescribed. When interpreting drug levels, the impact of acquired tolerance to drugs must be considered. Thus, death may result from very low levels of a drug in someone who has not developed tolerance to it. In postmortem toxicology the question is usually accidental overdose of a prescribed medication or suicidal overdosing on the drug. To this one may add toxic effects or sudden death due to polymorphisms at the receptor or enzyme level. In many cases measurement of parent drug to metabolite ratios is useful, followed by pharmacogenomic testing if variant alleles are known to be involved as a risk factor. Thus, a high ratio between codeine and morphine could suggest acute ingestion (attempted suicide), or that the person is a poor metabolizer. In an ultrametabolizer the ratio would be reversed.[28]

PHARMACOGENOMIC DATABASES

Table 8 provides the available pharmacogenomic databases that may be useful to the clinical laboratory. In this review, owing to the ever changing nature of pharmacogenomic data, we have not tried to exhaustively discuss every CYP gene/drug combination that may be useful in a toxicological setting. Rather our intention is to introduce the user to the key pharmacogenomic data bases and provide a sampling of the type of information that may be gleaned from them using *CYP2D6* and other genes as an example.

The cypalleles.ki.se Database

The Human Cytochrome P450 (CYP) Allele Nomenclature Web site is a peer-reviewed database of CYP variants and their associated effects (**Table 9**). Currently, this Web

Table 7
Pharmacogenomic studies in postmortem specimens

Gene	Drug	Description	References
CYP2D6	Codeine	Large variation in morphine (M) to codeine (C) ratios. CYP2D6 genotyping suggested with unusually high or low M/C ratios.	Frost et al[28]
CYP2D6	Methadone	CYP2D6 mutations may not be directly associated with methadone toxicity.	Wong et al[29]
CYP2D6	Oxycodone	Genotyping can be useful in some cases of oxycodone toxicity.	Jannetto et al[30]
CYP2D6	Tramadol	Correlation between number of functional CYP2D6 alleles to drug/metabolite ratios.	Levo et al[31]
CYP3A4*1B CYP3A5*3	Fentanyl	Homozygous CYP3A5 causes impaired metabolism of fentanyl. Fetanyl to nor-fentanyl ratios were abnormal.	Jin et al[32]
CYP2D6	Hydrocodone	Fatal overdose in a CYP2D6*41 carrier	Madadi et al[33]
ABCB1/MDR1	Digoxin	Link between ABCB1 SNPs and mortality due to digoxin.	Neuvonen et al[34]
CYP2D6 CYP2C19	Amitryptyline	Six metabolites were analyzed. Correlation between trans-hydroxylated metabolites and number of functional copies of CYP2D6 and demethylated metabolites and functional copies of CYP2C19.	Koski et al[35]

site covers the nomenclature for polymorphic alleles of 22 CYP isoforms including more than 200 functionally different variants. Each CYP has its own Web page, which lists the alleles with their nucleotide changes, their functional consequences, and links to publications where the allele has been identified and characterized. The CYP allele Web site offers a rapid on-line publication of new alleles, provides an overview of peer-reviewed data, and serves as a form of quality control on research on new alleles. For any CYP allele (written in italicized letters), the protein/enzyme name, the nucleotide changes, restriction fragment size, effect on enzyme activity, and relevant methodological references can be obtained. In the above listed example for the CYP2D6*2XN gene, N represents the copy number of duplicated CYP2D6 alleles and CYP2D6.2 is the corresponding protein (written according to standard nomenclature in nonitalicized letters). In addition, the database lists three nucleotide variations that have been identified in these alleles (eg, 1661 G>C, guanine replaced by cytosine at position 1661), corresponding to Arg-296-→ Cys (protein changes are denoted by the

Table 8
Key resources for pharmacogenomic data

Topic	Description	Website
Human cytochrome P450 database	Catalog of CYP450 genes, allelic variants, and related links	www.cypalleles.ki.se
FINDbase	Allele frequencies of inherited defects and ethnic and racial variation	www.findbase.org
PharmGKB	Curated pharmacogenomic data	www.pharmgkb.org

Table 9
Sample data from the cypalleles.ki.se database

Allele	Protein	Nucleotide Changes	Xbal Haplotype (kb)	Trivial Name	Effect	Enzyme Activity in Vivo or in Vitro	References
CYP2D6*2XN (N = 2, 3, 4, 5 or 13)	CYP2D6.2	1661G>C; 2850C>T; 4180G>C	42–175		R296C; S486T; N active genes	Incr (d)[39]	Johansson et al[36], Aklillu et al[37], Dahl et al[38]

Abbreviation: d, debrisoquine.

one-letter amino acid code). These alleles can be identified using the restriction enzyme *Xba*1 that generates restriction fragment sizes of 42 to 175 kb by pulsed field gel electrophoresis.[36–38] These amino acid changes result in increased activity of the enzyme debrisoquine (d).[39] SNPs 2850C>T and 4180G>C have been previously described. Clicking on SNP 2850 C>T, for example, leads to the SNP database of the National Center for Biotechnology Information (NCBI) (http://www.ncbi.nlm.nih.gov/SNP), providing information about the SNP position of the polymorphism in the *CYP2D6* gene as well as access to the ALFRED[40] (Allele Frequency Data Base), which specifies the worldwide distribution of the queried allele (**Fig. 2**).

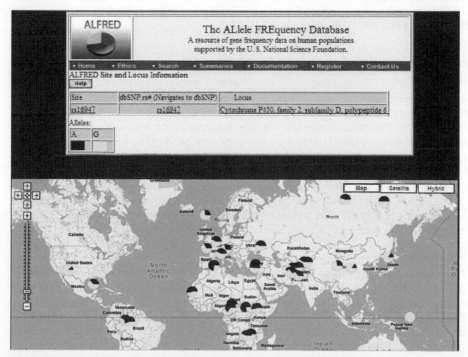

Fig. 2. The ALFRED database piecharts showing worldwide allele frequency distribution. (*From* http://alfred.med.yale.edu/. Accessed August 8, 2012.)

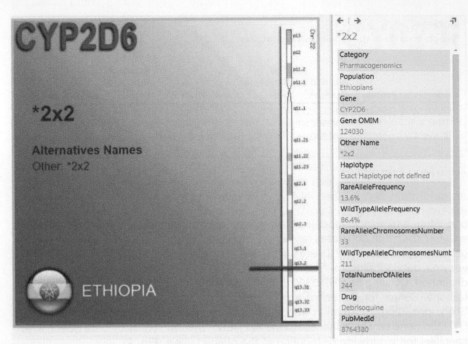

Fig. 3. Snapshot from the FINDBASE.org database, which shows the allele name, geographic location, ethnicity, and the rare allele frequency. It also shows the genetic location of *CYP2D6* on chromosome 22. (*From* van Baal S, Kaimakis P, Phommarinh M, et al. FINDbase: a relational database recording frequencies of genetic defects leading to inherited disorders worldwide. Nucleic Acids Res 2007;35[Database issue]:D690–5.)

Findbase.org Database—Genome Variation Allele Frequencies Worldwide

FINDbase is an online resource[41] documenting frequencies of pathogenic genetic variations leading to inherited disorders in various populations worldwide. This information is available in two separate modules: Causative mutations and Pharmacogenomic markers. The Pharmacogenomics module documents the frequency of pharmacogenomically relevant SNPs, based on ethnicity and geographic location worldwide. It also provides the rare allele frequencies as well as links to Online Mendelian Inheritance in Man (OMIM) and the PharmGKB entries. Thus, for example, using the FINDbase, Pharmacogenomics module, one can see that the rare allele frequency of CYP2D6 *2 × 2 duplication in Ethiopians is 13.6%. This pharmacogenomics database continues to expand, and is as yet not very comprehensive in relation to CYP gene polymorphisms (see **Fig. 3**).

The PharmGKb Database

The PharmGKb data base PGRN is supported by the National Institutes of Health, U.S. Department of Health and Human Services. The pgrn.org Web site is managed by the PharmGKB. This database[42] is quite extensive and has a wealth of information. With respect to *CYP2D6*, it describes the gene variants and the major therapeutic drugs that are relevant to the gene variants. The role of the CYP enzymes in drug metabolism is explained, and as an example the curated metabolic pathway for codeine and morphine by CYP enzymes is shown above (see **Fig. 1**). It also discusses genetic testing of *CYP2D6* alleles, using microarray-based technologies.

QUALITY ASSURANCE ISSUES IN PGX TESTING

Although numerous laboratories are now offering pharmacogenetic testing, there are major challenges associated with the implementation of these tests in clinical practice. These include clinical validation and reliability of genotyping, access to testing, uniformity and clarity in test interpretation, and clinician and patient education, which are critical to this process of innovation diffusion. Moreover, unlike many heritable disease mutations, each pharmacogenetic allele may include several SNPs, rather than a single-site mutation, requiring analysis of numerous mutations rather than individual ones. The Pharmacogenetic nomenclature further adds to the analytic and reporting complexity, especially when trying to compare various assay platforms. Another challenge is the availability of characterized quality control material to ensure quality of testing and provide reference material for test development, validation, quality control, and proficiency testing. To address these needs, recently the Centers for Disease Control and Prevention (CDC)-based Genetic Testing Reference Material Coordination Program (GeT-RM, http://wwwn.cdc.gov/dls/genetics/rmmaterials/default.aspx), in collaboration with the Association for Molecular Pathology, members of the pharmacogenetic testing community, and the Coriell Cell Repositories (Camden, NJ, USA), have characterized a panel of 107 genomic DNA reference material for five loci (*CYP2D6*, *CYP2C19*, *CYP2C9*, *VKORC1*, and *UGT1A1*) commonly included in pharmacogenetic testing panels and proficiency testing surveys.

FUTURE DIRECTIONS IN PHARMACOGENETIC TESTING

Current genetic testing approaches rely on targeting individual genetic variations in candidate genes. These genetic approaches typically target the more common SNPs prevalent in the Caucasian population, excluding other population such as people of African ancestry who are more difficult to tag. The completion of the Human Genome Project, The International HapMap Consortium, and the 1000 Genome Project Consortium, together with the availability of new high-throughput sequencing technologies, offers new opportunities for personalized medicine and individualized drug therapy in pharmacogenomics. New techniques such as whole genome, exome, and transcriptome sequencing at the individual level will allow identification of rare or uncommon gene variations regardless of the ethnic origin. Interestingly, it is thought that variants with stronger effects will be rare as they may be more deleterious at a population level. The complexity of data handling and analysis will be a major difficulty to overcome, and new and improved bioinformatics analyses tools as well strong databases will be required for analyzing the pathogenic potential of variants of uncertain significance. Finally, clinical implementation of such testing will also require the development of new standards and guidelines for testing, as well as major support from regulatory agencies such as the FDA and Centers for Medicare & Medicaid Services.

REFERENCES

1. Weinshilboum RM, Wang L. Pharmacogenetics and pharmacogenomics: development, science, and translation. Annu Rev Genomics Hum Genet 2006;7:223–45.
2. Linder MW, Valdes R Jr. Pharmacogenetics in the practice of laboratory medicine. Mol Diagn 1999;4:365–79.
3. Swen JJ, Nijenhuis M, de Boer A, et al. Pharmacogenetics: from bench to byte — an update of guidelines. Clin Pharmacol Ther 2011;89:662–73.

4. Becquemont L, Alfirevic A, Amstutz U, et al. Practical recommendations for pharma-cogenomics-based prescription: 2010 ESF-UB Conference on Pharmacogenetics and Pharmacogenomics. Pharmacogenomics 2011;12:113–24.

5. Amstutz U, Carleton BC. Pharmacogenetic testing: time for clinical practice guide-lines. Clin Pharmacol Ther 2011;89:924–7.

6. Scott SA. Personalizing medicine with clinical pharmacogenetics. Genet Med 2011; 13:987–95.

7. Johnson JA, Gong L, Whirl-Carrillo M, et al. Clinical Pharmacogenetics Implementa-tion Consortium Guidelines for CYP2C9 and VKORC1 genotypes and warfarin dos-ing. Clin Pharmacol Ther 2011;90:625–9.

8. Chan A, Pirmohamed M, Comabella M. Pharmacogenomics in neurology: current state and future steps. Ann Neurol 2011;70:684–97.

9. Roden DM, Johnson JA, Kimmel SE, et al. Cardiovascular pharmacogenomics. Circ Res 2011;109:807–20.

10. Ma Q, Lu AY. Pharmacogenetics, pharmacogenomics, and individualized medicine. Pharmacol Rev 2011;63:437–59.

11. U.S. Food and Drug Administration. Table of pharmacogenomic biomarkers in drug labels. Available at: http://www.fda.gov/drugs/scienceresearch/researchareas/pharmacogenetics/ucm083378.htm. Accessed April 9, 2012.

12. Johansson I, Ingelman-Sundberg M. Genetic polymorphism and toxicology—with emphasis on cytochrome p450. Toxicol Sci 2011;120:1–13.

13. Amstutz U, Carleton BC. Pharmacogenetic testing: time for clinical practice guide-lines. Clin Pharmacol Ther 2011;89:924–7.

14. Ingelman-Sundberg M, Daly AK, Nebert DW, et al, editors. The Human Cytochrome P450 (CYP) Allele Nomenclature Database. Available at: www.cypalleles.ki.se. Ac-cessed August 8, 2012.

15. Substance Abuse and Mental Health Services Administration, Drug Abuse Warning Network, 2009. National Estimates of Drug-Related Emergency Department Visits. HHS Publication No. (SMA) 11-4659, DAWN Series D-35. Rockville (MD): Substance Abuse and Mental Health Services Administration, 2011. Available at: http://www.samhsa.gov/data/2k11/DAWN/2k9DAWNED/HTML/DAWN2k9ED.htm. Accessed August 8, 2012.

16. Bissell MG, Peat MA. In: Magnani BJ, Bissell MG, Kwong TC, et al, editors. Clinical toxicology testing: a guide for laboratory professionals. Northfield (IL): CAP Press; 2012. p. 140–7.

17. Smith HS. Opioid metabolism. Mayo Clin Proc 2009;84:613–24.

18. Crews KR, Gaedigk A, Dunnenberger HM, et al and Clinical Pharmacogenetics Implementation Consortium. Clinical Pharmacogenetics Implementation Consortium (CPIC) guidelines for codeine therapy in the context of cytochrome P450 2D6 (CYP2D6) genotype. Clin Pharmacol Ther 2012;91:321–6.

19. Meyer MR, Maurer HH. Absorption, distribution, metabolism and excretion pharma-cogenomics of drugs of abuse. Pharmacogenomics 2011;12:215–33.

20. Maurer HH, Sauer C, Theobald DS. Toxicokinetics of drugs of abuse: current knowledge of the isoenzymes involved in the human metabolism of tetrahydrocan-nabinol, cocaine, heroin, morphine, and codeine. Ther Drug Monit 2006;28:447–53.

21. Levo A, Koski A, Ojanperä I, et al. Post-mortem SNP analysis of CYP2D6 gene reveals correlation between genotype and opioid drug (tramadol) metabolite ratios in blood. Forensic Sci Int 2003;135:9–15.

22. Jannetto PJ, Bratanow NC. Pain management in the 21st century: utilization of pharmacogenomics and therapeutic drug monitoring. Expert Opin Drug Metab Toxi-col 2011;7:745–52.

23. Lippi G, Plebani M. Pharmacogenomics of alcohol metabolism: implications for legal testing. Clin Chem Lab Med 2011;49:9–11.
24. Skopp G. Preanalytic aspects in postmortem toxicology. Forensic Sci Int 2004;142:75–100.
25. Skopp G. Postmortem toxicology. Forensic Sci Med Pathol 2010;6:314–25.
26. Drummer OH. Postmortem toxicology of drugs of abuse. Forensic Sci Int 2004;142:101–13.
27. Sajantila A, Palo JU, Ojanperä I, et al. Pharmacogenetics in medico-legal context. Forensic Sci Int 2010;203:44–52.
28. Frost J, Helland A, Nordrum IS, et al. Investigation of morphine and morphine glucuronide levels and cytochrome P450 isoenzyme 2D6 genotype in codeine-related deaths. Forensic Sci Int 2012;220(1–3):6–11.
29. Wong SH, Wagner MA, Jentzen JM, et al. Pharmacogenomics as an aspect of molecular autopsy for forensic pathology/toxicology: does genotyping CYP 2D6 serve as an adjunct for certifying methadone toxicity? J Forensic Sci 2003;48:1406–15.
30. Jannetto PJ, Wong SH, Gock SB, et al. Pharmacogenomics as molecular autopsy for postmortem forensic toxicology: genotyping cytochrome P450 2D6 for oxycodone cases. J Anal Toxicol 2002;26:438–47.
31. Levo A, Koski A, Ojanperä I, et al. Post-mortem SNP analysis of CYP2D6 gene reveals correlation between genotype and opioid drug (tramadol) metabolite ratios in blood. Forensic Sci Int 2003;135:9–15.
32. Jin M, Gock SB, Jannetto PJ, et al. Pharmacogenomics as molecular autopsy for forensic toxicology: genotyping cytochrome P450 3A4*1B and 3A5*3 for 25 fentanyl cases. J Anal Toxicol 2005;29:590–8.
33. Madadi P, Ross CJ, Hayden MR, et al. Pharmacogenetics of neonatal opioid toxicity following maternal use of codeine during breastfeeding: a case-control study. Clin Pharmacol Ther 2009;85:31–5.
34. Neuvonen AM, Palo JU, Sajantila A. Post-mortem ABCB1 genotyping reveals an elevated toxicity for female digoxin users. Int J Legal Med 2011;125:265–9.
35. Koski A, Sistonen J, Ojanperä I, et al. CYP2D6 and CYP2C19 genotypes and amitriptyline metabolite ratios in a series of medicolegal autopsies. Forensic Sci Int 2006;158:177–83.
36. Johansson I, Lundqvist E, Bertilsson L, et al. Inherited amplification of an active gene in the cytochrome P450 CYP2D locus as a cause of ultrarapid metabolism of debrisoquine. Proc Natl Acad Sci U S A 1993;90:11825–9.
37. Aklillu E, Persson I, Bertilsson L, et al. Frequent distribution of ultrarapid metabolizers of debrisoquine in an Ethiopian population carrying duplicated and multiduplicated functional CYP2D6 alleles. J Pharmacol Exp Ther 1996;278:441–6.
38. Dahl ML, Johansson I, Bertilsson L, et al. Ultrarapid hydroxylation of debrisoquine in a Swedish population: analysis of the molecular genetic basis. J Pharmacol Exp Ther 1995;274:516–20.
39. Mahgoub A, Idle JR, Dring LG, et al. Polymorphic hydroxylation of debrisoquine in man. Lancet 1977;2:584–6.
40. Allele Frequency database. Available at: http://alfred.med.yale.edu/. Accessed August 8, 2012.
41. van Baal S, Kaimakis P, Phommarinh M, et al. FINDbase: a relational database recording frequencies of genetic defects leading to inherited disorders worldwide. Nucleic Acids Res 2007;35[Database issue]:D690–5.
42. Pharmacogenomics Knowledge Base. Available at: www.pharmgkb.org. Accessed August 8, 2012.

Regulatory Issues in Accreditation of Toxicology Laboratories

Michael G. Bissell, MD, PhD, MPH[a,b,*]

KEYWORDS

- CLIA '88 • CAP FUDT • ABFT/LAP • ASCLD/LAB • SAMHSA NLCP

KEY POINTS

- In the United States, the type of laboratory accreditation required by a toxicology laboratory depends on the purpose of the laboratory's testing menu: clinical versus forensic.
- Like all clinical laboratories, clinical toxicology laboratories are subject to direct federal regulatory requirements for Clinical Laboratory Improvement Amendments of 1988 (CLIA) certification, classified as waived, moderate, or high-complexity testing operations.
- CLIA requirements include on-site inspections and acceptable participation in proficiency testing, which may be met by achieving accreditation from an agency with CLIA-deemed status.
- Forensic toxicology laboratories are CLIA-exempt under federal regulations but nonetheless subject to all applicable state and local regulatory requirements, which typically mandate independent laboratory accreditation.
- Such accreditation is provided by the College of American Pathologists, American Board of Forensic Toxicology, American Society of Crime Lab Directors, and Substance Abuse and Mental Health Services Administration National Laboratory Certification Program.

Clinical toxicology laboratories, free-standing or hospital/clinic-based, and forensic toxicology laboratories, operate in a highly regulated environment. An attempt is made here to outline major US legal/regulatory issues and requirements relevant to accreditation of toxicology laboratories (state and local regulations are not covered in any depth). The most fundamental regulatory distinction to be made involves the purposes for which the laboratory operates: clinical vs non-clinical. The applicable

Disclosure: The author is the current chair of the College of American Pathologists' Toxicology Resource Committee, which oversees all CAP proficiency testing in toxicology and therapeutic drug monitoring.
[a] Department of Pathology, The Ohio State University, 4173 Graves Hall, 333 West 10th Avenue, Columbus OH 43210, USA; [b] Wexner Medical Center at the Ohio State University, 4173 Graves Hall, 333 West 10th Avenue, Columbus, OH 43210, USA
* Department of Pathology, The Ohio State University, 4173 Graves Hall, 313 West 10th Avenue, Columbus, OH 43210.
E-mail address: Michael.Bissell@osumc.edu

regulations and the requirements and options for operations depend most basically upon this consideration, with clinical toxicology laboratories being directly subject to federal law (CLIA) including mandated options for accreditation and forensic toxicology laboratories being subject to degrees of voluntary or state government-required accreditation.

CLINICAL LABORATORIES
CLIA Certification

All clinical laboratories in the United States performing testing on human specimens for purposes of diagnosis, treatment, or clinical management of patients operate under direct federal regulatory jurisdiction. With certain specific exceptions (outlined below) all US clinical laboratories are subject to the Clinical Laboratory Improvement Amendments of 1988 (CLIA or CLIA '88).[1] This set of regulations is aimed at dealing directly with the quality of laboratory results produced within its broad jurisdiction independent of reimbursement source or location nationwide (ie, the same regulations apply to laboratories operated on a commercial or nonprofit basis whether or not they receive any federal reimbursement—even though CLIA certification is required to qualify for such reimbursement).[2]

The CLIA definition of a *laboratory* is a "a facility for the biological, microbiological, serological, chemical, immunohematological, hematological, biophysical, cytological, pathological, or other examination of materials derived from the human body for the purpose of providing information for the diagnosis, prevention, or treatment of any disease or impairment of, or the assessment of the health of, human beings . . . . Facilities only collecting or preparing specimens (or both) or only serving as a mailing service and not performing testing are not considered laboratories."[3]

US clinical laboratories meeting this definition are universally classified under CLIA either as being CLIA-exempt or as performing waived or nonwaived testing[4]:

CLIA-Exempt Testing

CLIA-exempt laboratories include:
Nonclinical laboratories: Any facility or portion of a facility that performs testing on human specimens for purposes other than diagnosis, prevention, or treatment for individual patients, specifically those facilities engaged in testing such specimens for research or forensic (medicolegal) purposes, including workplace drug testing performed by Substance Abuse and Mental Health Services Administration (SAMHSA)-certified laboratories (although any other non-SAMHSA testing conducted by such laboratories is nonexempt).

Jurisdictional exemptions: Clinical laboratories under the jurisdiction of an agency of the federal government (specifically the military and Veterans' Administration), although generally subject to CLIA, may be exempted from portions of it by modifications enacted by the secretary of the Department of Health and Human Services (DHHS) as appropriate.

In addition, individual states can be exempt from CLIA 88 if they maintain clinical laboratory licensure programs determined by the Center for Medicare and Medicaid Services (CMS) to be equal to or more stringent than CLIA 88. To date, only Washington and New York have achieved this status.

The Washington State Office of Laboratory Quality Assurance, Washington Medical Test Site Licensure program provides several categories of licenses. Inspections are conducted by Department of Health Laboratory Quality Assurance surveyors or by one of the CLIA-deemed private accreditation organizations (see later).[5]

The New York State Department of Health operates a Clinical Laboratory Evaluation Program (CLEP) issuing annual operation permits to clinical laboratories and testing sites, both within and outside of the state, that produce results on specimens originating in New York. It also issues certificates of qualification (COQs) to individuals to serve as directors/assistant directors, conducts its own inspections, and maintains its own proficiency testing (PT) program.[6]

Waived Testing

The US Food and Drug Administration (FDA) is responsible for approving in vitro diagnostic test methods for human clinical use. Such approvals are further categorized by the FDA as being of waived, moderate, or high complexity for purposes of CLIA. A *waived test* must "employ methodologies that are so simple and accurate as to render the likelihood of erroneous results negligible" or "pose no reasonable risk of harm to the patient if the test is performed incorrectly."[7] Under the current process, waiver may be granted to (1) any test listed in the regulation, (2) any test system for which the manufacturer or producer applies for waiver if that test meets the statutory criteria and the manufacturer provides scientifically valid data verifying that the waiver criteria have been met, and (3) test systems cleared by the FDA for home use. A current list of waived test methods is maintained by FDA and can be found at the FDA website.[8] Several immunochemical drug screen devices are FDA classified as waived test methods.

A CLIA *certificate of waiver* allows a laboratory to perform waived testing only (ie, to use only test systems that are classified as waived by the FDA). The waived status is voided if users deviate from the manufacturer's directions. The manufacturer's directions must be followed and documented in records and worksheets to remain in compliance. Waived testing does not require PT (described later). A health care facility may elect to establish a "waived lab" with a certificate of waiver that is organizationally distinct from its clinical laboratory, especially if the clinical laboratory director is not responsible for this testing. Although a waived laboratory is subject to announced or unannounced inspections, none are performed on a regularly scheduled basis.

Nonwaived Testing

For laboratories seeking full accreditation for nonwaived testing, CLIA requires 5 categories of compliance and documentation, known as "condition level requirements": namely: participation in PT, facility administration, quality systems, personnel, and inspection.

PT

Successful ongoing participation in PT by enrollment in a CMS-approved PT program is required for analytes listed individually in the CLIA 88 regulation and analyzed by nonwaived methods (known as the "regulated analytes").[9] For toxicology/therapeutic drug monitoring (TDM), the regulated analytes include blood alcohol, blood lead, and the following therapeutic drugs in serum, plasma, or blood:

- Carbamazepine
- Digoxin
- Ethosuximide
- Gentamicin
- Lithium
- Phenobarbital
- Phenytoin

- Primidone
- Procainamide (and metabolite)
- Quinidine
- Theophylline
- Tobramycin
- Valproic acid.

The frequency for this required PT is 5 specimen challenges on each of 3 PT events per year, of which 80% of challenges on 2 of 3 consecutive events must be reported within a specified range of the target value established by the PT program, for the laboratory to achieve successful participation.[9] The acceptable range is:

a. +25% for blood alcohol, carbamazepine, gentamicin, phenytoin, primidone, procainamide/NAPA, quinidine, tobramycin, theophylline, and valproic acid
b. +20% for ethosuximide and phenobarbital
c. The greater of +20% OR +0.2 ng/mL for digoxin and +20% OR +0.3 mmol/L for lithium
d. The greater of +10% OR +4 µg/dL for blood lead.

PT of the nonregulated analytes, including drugs of abuse and therapeutic drugs in matrices other than serum, plasma, or blood, is not required by CMS. The College of American Pathologists (CAP) and other programs with deemed status for CLIA accreditation (see later) specify the PT programs approved for their accreditation programs, including most nonregulated analytes.

CMS maintains a list of approved PT providers.[10] For regulated and nonregulated analytes of interest in toxicology, PT providers of nationwide scope among these include the American Association for Clinical Chemistry (AACC) (in conjunction with CAP), the American College of Physicians (ACP) Medical Laboratory Evaluation program (MLE), the American Proficiency Institute (API), CAP, and the Wisconsin State Laboratory of Hygiene (WSLH). PT programs of more limited scope include the New York State Department of Health Wadsworth Center's routine drug testing PT module for laboratories holding New York State clinical laboratory permits and PT provided by the Substance Abuse and Mental Health Services Administration (SAMHSA) for toxicology laboratories accredited under its National Laboratory Certification Program (NCLP).

Facility administration
This includes providing space, ventilation, utilities, minimization of contamination, appropriate and sufficient equipment, instruments, reagents, materials, and supplies for the testing performed, as well as laboratory safety and record retention.[11]

Laboratory safety procedures must be established, accessible, and observed to ensure protection from physical, chemical, biochemical, and electrical hazards, and biohazardous materials. In addition to CLIA, there are several Occupational Safety and Health Administration (OSHA) and other federal, state, and local regulations and guidelines that require safety compliance. These include OSHA standards for air contaminants – permissible exposure limits,[12] general housekeeping requirements,[13] hazard communication,[14] occupational exposure to bloodborne pathogens,[15] occupational exposure to hazardous chemicals in laboratories,[16] occupational injury and illness recording and reporting,[17] personal protective equipment,[18] sanitation and waste disposal,[19] and specifications for accident prevention signs and tags.[20] Under the Medical Waste Tracking Act of 1988: Standards for the Tracking and Management of Medical Waste[21] and updated US Public Health Service guidelines for the management of occupational exposures to hepatitis B virus, hepatitis C virus, and human immunodeficiency virus and recommendations for postexposure prophylaxis.

Laboratory records are subject to the Health Insurance Portability and Accountability Act of 1996[22] and subsequent regulations that include protected health information (confidentiality) and electronic medical records (EMRs). The records retention requirements for toxicology are that test requisitions and authorizations, test procedures (standard operating procedures [SOP]), analytic systems records including quality control, patient test records and instrument printouts, records of test system performance, PT records, quality system assessment records, and test reports are all required to be retained for 2 years (the period between on-site inspections, see later).[23] Retention in electronic format is acceptable providing they can be printed in their original format as appropriate. These record retention requirements are minimum for accreditation, but other considerations may also apply to determining how long records should be retained. For instance, the laboratory compliance plan and the potential for audits by the Office of the Inspector General or DHHS may necessitate longer retention of certain records such as state or other accrediting agency requirements. The most stringent of the applicable requirements should be followed.

Quality systems

According to CLIA: "Each laboratory that performs nonwaived testing must establish and maintain written policies and procedures that implement and monitor a quality system for all phases of the total testing process (that is, preanalytic, analytic, and postanalytic) as well as general laboratory systems." "This must include a quality assessment component that ensures continuous improvement of the laboratory's performance and services through ongoing monitoring that identifies, evaluates and resolves problems."[24]

Quality assessment must include documented policies and procedures for general laboratory systems quality assessment including test requisition, specimen submission, handling, and referral, procedure manual, test systems, equipment, instruments, reagents, materials, supplies, method performance specifications and validation, maintenance and function checks, calibration and calibration verification, control procedures, comparison of same test results when different methodologies, instruments or sites are used, corrective actions, test records, analytic systems assessment, and test report.

The toxicology service in a hospital or clinic setting must be included in the laboratory's overall quality assessment/quality management plan. Items of special interest to the toxicology laboratory include patient and specimen identification, internal and external chain of custody documents (if created), interpretation of analytic data, scientific review of data, and accurate reporting as appropriate to the specific laboratory. Chromatography and mass spectral methods require a significant amount of interpretation and attention to reporting and are appropriate topics for assessment.

Proficiency testing and alternative performance assessment Most clinical toxicology tests are not CLIA-regulated analytes, but CLIA requires verification of their accuracy at least twice per year. This requirement can be met or exceeded by participating in PT when available through a CLIA-approved provider. Alternative performance assessment is required for those tests for which there is no appropriate PT program or if the accrediting organization does not require PT for nonregulated analytes. Appropriate alternative performance assessment procedures may include participation in ungraded PT programs, split sample analysis with reference or other laboratories, split samples with an established in-house method, assayed material, regional pools, clinical validation by chart review, or other suitable and documented means.[25]

Evaluation and corrective action of unsatisfactory PT and alternative performance assessments are required for both regulated and nonregulated analytes. The laboratory director is responsible for the method of assessment. There must be evidence of laboratory director or designee review of PT reports including the cause of the unsatisfactory result, the corrective action taken, and an evaluation of whether patient results could have been effected and, if so, the course of action taken. Results not graded, not submitted on time, or not submitted at all also need evaluation. These evaluations and corrective actions must be documented and reviewed by the laboratory director or designee.

Method validation Many toxicology methods are locally implemented "home brew procedures" based on scientific literature but without formal FDA clearance status (ie, so-called laboratory developed tests [LDTs]). These include most gas chromatography, liquid chromatography, and mass spectral methods, which, as LDTs, require validation of the entire testing process including applicability, accuracy, precision, interfering substances, cross-reactivity, reportable range of results, dilution protocol, reference intervals, calibration, and control procedures. The laboratory director is responsible for determining the method of validation. The FDA has recently indicated interest in more directly regulating home brew methods so the laboratory needs to stay current on relevant regulatory developments in this area.

Personnel

CLIA regulations provide qualifications and responsibilities for laboratory director, technical consultant, clinical consultant, technical supervisor, general supervisor, and testing personnel. The qualification requirements and responsibilities are quite detailed and specific. In general, as noted earlier, for most CLIA purposes, the FDA classification of test methods into "waived," "moderate complexity," and "high complexity," based on the skill level demanded by each procedure, has been collapsed into the simple distinction between "waived" and "nonwaived" testing. The one exception to this is in the section on personnel, in which the experiential and/or educational qualifications for each category of worker in nonwaived laboratories are different for laboratories performing "moderate complexity" versus "high complexity" testing. So, for example, laboratory directors with a doctorate who began directing high complexity testing after February 24, 2003, must be certified by an approved board, unlike those directing labs of only moderate complexity; and, in order that their work not require daily review, testing personnel in high complexity settings must have an educational background including course work equivalent to an associate degree in clinical laboratory sciences, unlike their colleagues in moderate complexity settings.

The 15 responsibilities of CLIA laboratory directors[26] include ensuring that:
a. Testing systems provide quality laboratory services for all aspects of test performance (preanalytic, analytic, and postanalytic).
b. Physical plant and environmental conditions of the laboratory are appropriate and safe.
c. Test methodologies provide quality results required for patient care; accuracy, precision, and other pertinent performance characteristics are verified; and laboratory personnel are properly performing the test methods as required.
d. PT samples are tested as required; PT results are returned within the timeframes established by the PT program; all PT reports received are reviewed by the

appropriate staff to evaluate the laboratory's performance and to identify any problems that require corrective action; and an approved corrective action plan is followed when any PT failures occur.

e. Quality control and quality assessment programs are established and maintained to assure the quality of laboratory services provided and to identify quality control failures as they occur.

f. Acceptable levels of analytical performance for each test system are established and maintained.

g. All necessary remedial actions are taken and documented whenever significant deviations from the laboratory's established performance characteristics are identified, and that patient test results are reported only when the system is functioning properly.

h. Reports of test results include pertinent information required for interpretation.

i. Consultation is available to the laboratory's clients on matters relating to the quality of the test results reported and their interpretation concerning specific patient conditions.

j. A general supervisor provides on-site supervision of high complexity test performance by qualified testing personnel.

k. A sufficient number of laboratory personnel with the appropriate education and either experience or training are employed to provide appropriate consultation, supervision, performance and reporting of tests in accordance with CLIA requirements.

l. Prior to testing patients' specimens, all personnel have the appropriate education and experience, receive the appropriate training for the type and complexity of the services offered, and have demonstrated that they can perform all testing operations reliably to provide and report accurate results.

m. Policies and procedures are established for monitoring individuals who conduct preanalytical, analytical, and postanalytical phases of testing to ensure that they are competent and maintain their competency to process specimens, perform test procedures and report test results promptly and proficiently, and, whenever necessary, provide needs for remedial training or continuing education to improve skills.

n. An approved procedure manual is available to all personnel responsible for any aspect of the testing process.

o. Responsibilities and duties of each consultant and each supervisor, as well as each person engaged in the performance of testing are spelled out that identify which examinations and procedures each individual is authorized to perform, whether supervision is required for specimen processing, test performance or result reporting and whether supervisory or director review is required prior to reporting patient test results.

[Note that responsibilities c, d, e, f, g, l, m, and n can be delegated in writing to a technical supervisor and h and i to a clinical consultant, but a, b, j, k, and o cannot be delegated.]

Competency evaluation of technical staff must be performed at 6 months, 12 months, and annually thereafter. Note that this evaluation may be more involved with confirmatory tests in toxicology involving extraction, chromatography and mass spectrometry, and interpreting results. There are 6 required components of such evaluations[27]:

a. Directly observing routine patient test performance, including patient preparation, if applicable, specimen handling, processing, and testing.

b. Monitoring recording and reporting of test results.

c. Reviewing intermediate test results or worksheets, quality control records, PT results, and preventive maintenance records.
d. Directly observing performance of instrument maintenance and function.
e. Assessing test performance through testing previously analyzed specimens, internal blind testing samples, or external PT samples.
f. Assessing problem-solving skills.

Inspection

All CLIA-certified nonwaived laboratories require an on-site inspection every 2 years performed by CMS personnel or by an agent of CMS (eg, a state program inspector, the licensure department of a CLIA-exempt state [New York and Washington]) or by one of the nongovernmental organizations (NGOs) (private, nonprofit accreditation programs) granted "deemed status" by CMS for CLIA accreditation.

CMS is authorized under CLIA to grant this deemed status to private nonprofit accreditation agencies whose requirements are judged to be are equal to or more stringent than those of CLIA after an extensive review process including CMS-performed validation reinspections. Currently, organizations with deemed status for CLIA include the CAP, The Joint Commission (TJC; formerly, the Joint Commission for the Accreditation of Healthcare Organizations [JCAHO]), the Committee on Office Laboratory Accreditation (COLA), the American Osteopathic Association (AOA), the American Association of Blood Banks (AABB), and the American Society for Histo-compatibility and Immunogenetics (ASHI). [The AABB and ASHI programs are focused on specific subdisciplines only.]

A CLIA *certificate of registration* issued by CMS is required for a new laboratory to begin performing waived or nonwaived testing until they receive a certificate of waiver or certificate of accreditation. It is also required for a laboratory testing under a certificate of waiver that begins nonwaived testing. A CLIA *certificate of compliance* is issued after an inspection by CMS or governmental agent thereof that finds the laboratory to be in compliance with all applicable CLIA condition level requirements or a CLIA *certificate of accreditation* is issued by CMS on the basis of the laboratory's accreditation by one of the private nonprofit organizations with deemed status under CLIA listed earlier. CMS provides a certificate of compliance or accreditation only after any deficiencies cited during the inspection are corrected.

Additional inspections may be performed by CMS, CAP, or the agency or program that accredits the laboratory following a complaint or for other reasons. CMS or a CMS agent may also inspect a waived laboratory for complaints, to ensure that laboratory testing does not constitute an imminent and serious risk to public health, to determine whether the laboratory is performing tests beyond the scope of their certificate, and/or to collect information regarding the appropriateness of tests specified as waived. CMS or a CMS agent will perform a certain percentage of reinspections after inspections by CMS agents, CLIA-exempt programs, and those performed by deemed status programs for validation purposes.

FORENSIC TESTING AND FORENSIC LABORATORIES

Forensic toxicology testing can be broadly defined as non–clinical laboratory testing for drugs (abused and/or therapeutic), alcohol, or toxic agents that is conducted specifically for legal purposes. Such purposes may include pre-mortem workplace testing (either for preemployment screening or "for cause") or for law enforcement activities (eg, traffic violations, either "driving under the influence" of alcohol [DUI] or of drugs [DUID] or in connection with charges of use/possession of illegal substances). They may also include postmortem testing in cause-of-death investigations by coroner's and medical examiner's offices and testing of unknown substances seized as part of drug raids or crime scene investigations.

Clinical Testing with Legal Implications

It should be noted that virtually any or all clinical laboratory testing conducted in the course of screening, diagnosing, treating, or managing inpatients or outpatients, even though not strictly "forensic," may nonetheless have legal implications (either civil or criminal) at any time. Some of the more likely situations involving clinical toxicology testing might include drug testing of pregnant women, newborns, young children, and those involved in accidents. The laboratory may not be aware of it, but specimens and lab records from such cases may carry an enhanced likelihood of being subject to subpoena. Unless ordered by law enforcement or the judicial system, these are typically handled under clinical laboratory regulations (ie, treated as "medical" versus "legal" blood alcohols or drug screens). The decision about whether the laboratory elects to follow chain-of-custody and other forensic procedures with these specimens may be complex, since there is no regulatory requirement that they do so, and other hospital stakeholders' interests may be involved.

Of course, in addition, forensic drug testing (per se) may also be performed in the clinical laboratory. In such circumstances, it is advisable to have policies and procedures that clearly distinguish the medical from the forensic testing in day-to-day practice, separating forensic from clinical specimens in terms of location and/or timing of specimen handling and testing. CLIA does not include any requirements relevant to this; however, the CAP CHM inspection checklist does include a legal testing section that addresses forensic issues, including specimen collection, specimen containers, specimen receipt, accessioning, external and internal chain of custody, limited access, secure specimen storage, positive result confirmation, certifying review of chain-of-custody and testing data, confidentiality, specimen and record retention, ethanol specificity, and effect of lactate dehydrogenase and lactate on enzymatic ethanol methods.

Forensic Laboratory Accreditation

As noted earlier, toxicology laboratories performing only forensic testing are classified CLIA-exempt, so there are no federal accreditation requirements for these laboratories; however, some states and other jurisdictions have accreditation requirements that apply. (Of course, if a forensic testing laboratory also performs any clinical testing, it must be CLIA-certified for that testing.) Accreditation programs for forensic testing include the CAP Forensic Drug Testing accreditation program (CAP FDT, formerly FUDT [Forensic Urine Drug Testing Accreditation Program]),[28] the American Board of Forensic Toxicology Laboratory Accreditation Program (ABFT LAP),[29] and the American Society of Crime Laboratory Directors Laboratory Accreditation Board (ASCLD/LAB)[30] programs. Furthermore, workplace drug testing of certain federal employees under the SAMHSA regulations requires National Laboratory Certification Program (NLCP) certification.[31]

Broadly speaking, each of these programs has standards/requirements for accreditation that mirror the 5 "condition-level" requirements of CLIA (ie, participation in PT, facility administration, quality systems, personnel, and inspection) and has eligibility requirements as follows:

The CAP FDT Accreditation Program

a. *Eligibility:* Laboratories performing workplace drug testing of urine, oral fluid, or hair.

b. *PT*: The laboratory is required to participate in a PT system that covers the extent and complexity of analytical procedures and is CAP accepted. For tests that the CAP-accepted PT does not cover, the director must develop a mechanism for determining their reliability. The director must monitor the results of PT and participate in the documentation of corrective actions.

c. *Facilities*: There must be sufficient resources to provide immunoassay screening and quantitative mass spectral confirmation of positives: physical space, testing instruments, reagents, information processing and communication systems, refrigerated and freezer storage space, and storage and waste disposal facilities, ventilation, public utilities, safety, and accommodation for disability of employees. Access to all specimens, data, records, and reports must be restricted.

d. *Quality*: The laboratory must have policies and procedures to ensure quality laboratory testing and chain-of-custody documentation, including, but not limited to, validation of test systems, analytic quality control, quality management of preanalytic and postanalytic processes, PT (or periodic alternative assessments of laboratory test performance), human resource management, information management, ongoing quality improvement, and client communication.

e. *Personnel:* Qualifications for laboratory director/scientific director: board-certified pathologist or other qualified physician or qualified doctoral scientist or certification by the ABFT or certification in toxicological chemistry by the American Board of Clinical Chemistry. The director must have 2 years of active laboratory experience in analytical toxicology. For other personnel, the laboratory must be staffed with a sufficient number of personnel to perform quality laboratory testing.

f. *Inspections*: Laboratories will be evaluated in accordance with the CAP Standards for Laboratory Accreditation and the applicable version of the CAP Laboratory Accreditation Checklists, including biennial on-site inspection (conducted by peers with forensic experience), alternate-year self-assessment, and any interim inspections that the CAP Commission on Laboratory Accreditation (CLA) determines to conduct. When deficiencies are noted, corrective action shall be documented and subject to review by the CLA.[32]

ABFT Laboratory Accreditation Program

a. *Eligibility:* US or Canadian laboratories conducting either postmortem forensic toxicology or human performance toxicology (eg, DUID-type toxicology) or both, to include at least the detection, identification, and quantitation of alcohol and other drugs in biological specimens. Accreditation is for 1 year initially, with an extension given for a second year, subject to satisfactory review of a self-inspection checklist and of relevant proficiency test results for the 12 months following initial accreditation.

b. *PT:* Successful performance in the following 3 programs is required: CAP Whole Blood Alcohol, CAP Whole Blood Forensic Toxicology (FTC), **and** the CAP T-series.

   For both the CAP FTC and T-series programs, laboratories must perform qualitative screening and confirmation tests, as required, on all samples. Quantitative testing must be performed for all analytes that are included in the laboratory's list of routinely quantitated substances. For the T-series, quantitative testing may be limited to those analytes that the laboratory performs on a regular basis (defined as being within the reporting period set by CAP). "Acceptable performance" will be determined by the accreditation committee, based on the following: no false positives; ethanol within ± 2 SDs of the participant mean or $\pm 10\%$ weighed-in target; for drugs the challenges should be within ± 2 SDs of the participant mean or ±30% weighed-in target for drugs. Corrective action must be documented for false negatives and other deficiencies, appropriate for the stated mission of the laboratory. The accreditation committee may, in its discretion, accept proficiency test results outside these ranges if the laboratory can demonstrate that appropriate action has been taken and that the errors are not systematic and are unlikely to recur or if the target concentration of the analyte is very low.

c. *Facilities:* Access to the laboratory must be controlled during working hours, limited to authorized personnel with unauthorized personnel being escorted and required to sign a logbook upon entry and departure. The physical layout should provide adequate security insured with proper locks and key distribution being controlled. Monitoring devices and security personnel may also be necessary. Both long- and short-term specimen storage must have adequate space and be fully secured, and record storage areas must likewise be adequate and secure with access strictly restricted to authorized personnel.

d. *Quality:* The laboratory must maintain available external chain-of-custody, requisition, and/or shipping information, document all persons handling the specimens, with transfer and handling of specimens clearly documented as part of the permanent laboratory records and should indicate, at a minimum, the date and identity of the individuals involved in the specimen transfer and laboratory identification number. This document may be a logbook, worksheet, or other suitable means of recording the information.

e. *Personnel:* Required education and experience are outlined for laboratory director, who should be either a certified diplomate of the ABFT or hold a doctorate in a chemical or biological science with 3 years' full-time laboratory experience in forensic toxicology, a master's degree in a chemical or biological science with 5 years of such laboratory experience, or a bachelor's degree in a chemical or biological discipline with 7 years of laboratory experience in forensic toxicology. Full documentation of the director's qualifications must be maintained on site. The responsibilities of the laboratory director must include daily management of the laboratory, preparation and revision of the standard operating procedure manual, establishing procedures for validating new assays, maintaining a quality assurance program, and training laboratory staff.

There should be a person on staff with sufficient training and experience to substitute for the director in case of his or her absence. There must be sufficient personnel on staff for operations and these personnel have to be familiar with all areas of toxicologic testing within their responsibility and understand how their responsibilities relate to the operation of the laboratory as a whole. Training should include but not be limited to theory and practice of methods and procedures that the individual performs, understanding quality control practices and procedures, maintenance of chain of custody, laboratory safety, etc. The director is responsible for providing adequate training of personnel and for maintaining the competency of laboratory personnel by monitoring their work performance and verifying their skills. Records must be maintained to support the qualifications, experience, and training for all personnel. These records may either be maintained in an individual's personnel file or in separate training files, to include training checklists/summaries, resume, copies of certificates, copies of diplomas, copies of licenses, and testimony experience. Job descriptions must be available for all personnel. There must be a written policy on continuing education of personnel.

f. *Inspections:* The program cycle is 2 years. Laboratories must submit to an on-site inspection at least once every 2 years (normally 2 inspectors on site for 2 days, up to 3 inspectors on site for 3 days). Checklist questions are designated either essential, important, or desirable. All essential questions must be answerable "yes" before accreditation can be granted. The laboratory must also satisfy at least 90% of the important questions and at least 75% of the desirable questions. Areas of testing within the laboratory other than postmortem forensic toxicology or human performance toxicology will not be evaluated, unless there is overlap.[33]

ASCLD/LAB

a. *Eligibility:* Public and private crime laboratories and breath alcohol calibration laboratories in the United States and internationally (under International Organization for Standardization/International Electrotechnical Commission (ISO/IEC) 17025 2005).

b. *PT:* Toxicology is only one of the forensic disciplines covered by ASCLD/LAB accreditation, the others being such things as forensic biology/DNA, crime scene testing, drug analysis, trace evidence, firearms, latent prints, etc. Accredited labs are required to participate in an ASCLD-approved PT program for each forensic discipline they are engaged in. Approved PT providers for toxicology include collaborative testing services (CTS) for blood alcohol and breath alcohol and the CAP for its forensic toxicology (criminalistics) (FTC) and blood alcohol (AL1) surveys. PT results are to be released directly to ASCLD/LAB by the PT program.

c. *Facilities:* Requirements are specified in ISO/IEC 17025 2005: There must be effective separation between neighboring areas when the activities therein are incompatible. Environmental conditions should not adversely affect the required quality of tests. The laboratory should monitor, control, and record environmental conditions. Special attention should be paid to biologic sterility, dust, electromagnetic disturbances, radiation, humidity, electrical supply, temperature, sound, and vibration. Tests should be stopped when the environmental conditions are outside specified ranges; access to test and calibration areas should be limited to authorized people. This can be achieved through the use of pass cards.

d. *Quality:* Requirements are specified in ISO/IEC 17025 2005 including methods and procedures should be used within their scope, which must be clearly defined. The laboratory should have up-to-date instructions on the use of methods and equipment. If standard methods are available for a specific sample test, the most recent edition should be used. Deviations from standard methods or from otherwise agreed-on methods should be reported to the customer and their agreement obtained. When using standard methods, the laboratory should verify its competence to successfully run the standard method. This can be achieved through repeating 1 or 2 critical validation experiments and/or through running method specific quality control and/or proficiency test samples. Standard methods should also be validated if they are partly or fully out of the scope of the test requirement. Methods as published in literature or developed by the laboratory can be used but should be fully validated. Clients should be informed and agree to the selected method. Introduction of laboratory-developed methods should proceed according to a plan. The following parameters should be considered for validating in-house developed methods: limit of detection, limit of quantitation, accuracy, selectivity, linearity, repeatability and/or reproducibility, robustness, and linearity. Exact validation experiments should be relevant to samples and required information. Sometimes, standard and in-house validated methods need to be adjusted or changed to ensure continuing performance, in which case, the influence of such changes should be documented and, if appropriate, a new validation should be carried out. Validation includes specification of the requirements and scope, determination of the characteristics of the methods, appropriate testing to prove that the requirements can be fulfilled by using the method, and a statement on validity. The laboratory should have a procedure to estimate the uncertainty of measurement for calibrations and testing. For uncertainty estimation, the laboratory should identify all the components of uncertainty. Sources contributing to the uncertainty can include the reference materials used, the methods and equipment used for sampling and testing, environmental conditions, and personnel. Calculations used for data evaluation should be checked. This is best done during software and computer system validation. Data transfer accuracy should be checked. Computer software used for instrument control, data acquisition, processing, reporting, data transfer, archiving, and retrieval developed by or for a specific user should be validated. The suitability of the complete computer system for the intended use should also be validated. Any modification or configuration of a commercial computer system should be validated. Electronic data should be protected to ensure integrity and confidentiality of electronic records.

e. *Personnel:* Requirements are specified in ISO/IEC 17025 2005. Competence can come from education, experience, or training. Management should define and maintain tasks, job descriptions, and required skills for each job. Based on required skills and available qualifications, a training program should be developed and implemented for each employee. The effectiveness of the training should be evaluated. If the training is related to a specific test method, the trainee can demonstrate adequate qualification through successfully running a quality control or proficiency test sample. A statement from the trainee such as "I have read through the test procedure" is not enough. Management should authorize personnel to perform specific tasks, for example, to operate specific types of instruments, to issue test reports, to interpret specific test results, and to train or supervise other personnel. The date of this authorization should be recorded. The associated tasks should not be performed before the authorization date.

f. *Inspections:* The accreditation cycle is 5 years with an initial and follow-up on site assessments. Crime labs required by their state laws to be accredited before providing evidentiary testing can also participate in a 1-year preliminary accreditation (which must be followed up within 9 months with an application for full 5-year accreditation).[34,35]

SAMHSA NLCP

a. *Eligibility:* Laboratories that perform workplace drug testing on specimens collected by federal agencies. In addition to the federal agencies that use DHHS-certified laboratories to test specimens for their workplace drug testing programs, the Department of Transportation, the Department of Energy, and the Nuclear Regulatory Commission require the industries they regulate to use DHHS-certified laboratories for their workplace drug testing programs.

b. *PT:* The NCLP operates its own PT program through a private-sector contractor (RTI, Inc), which provides samples of various biologic matrices (urine, oral fluid, hair, sweat, serum) prepared with relevant drug analytes at appropriate concentrations for the analysis of drugs in human specimens. To become certified initially, an applicant laboratory must successfully test 3 rounds of PT samples before being initially inspected. To maintain certification, a laboratory must participate in and satisfy the requirements for the "maintenance" PT program, consisting of sets of PT samples sent to each laboratory on a quarterly basis. In addition, there is an

Agency Blind Sample Program with detailed performance requirements on blind samples.

c. *Facilities:* Laboratory facilities must comply with applicable provisions of any state licensure requirements and must have the capability, at the same laboratory premises, of performing initial and confirmatory tests for each drug or metabolite for which service is offered. Drug testing laboratories must be secure at all times. They must have in place sufficient security measures to control access to the premises and to ensure that no unauthorized personnel handle specimens or gain access to the laboratory processes or to areas where records are stored. Access to these secured areas must be limited to specifically authorized individuals whose authorization is documented. With the exception of personnel authorized to conduct inspections on behalf of federal agencies for which the laboratory is engaged in urine testing or on behalf of the secretary or emergency personnel (eg, firefighters and medical rescue teams), all authorized visitors and maintenance and service personnel must be escorted at all times. The laboratory must maintain a record that documents the dates, time of entry and exit, and purpose of entry of authorized visitors, maintenance, and service personnel accessing secured areas.

d. *Quality:* Laboratories must have a quality assurance program that encompasses all aspects of the testing process including, but not limited to, specimen acquisition, chain-of-custody, security and reporting of results, initial and confirmatory testing, certification of calibrators and controls, and validation of analytical procedures. Quality assurance procedures shall be designed, implemented, and reviewed to monitor the conduct of each step of the testing process. For quality control, each analytical run of specimens to be screened shall include sample(s) certified to contain no drug (ie, negative urine samples), positive control(s) fortified with drug or metabolite, at least one positive control with the drug or metabolite at or near the threshold (cutoff), and a sufficient number of calibrators to ensure and document the linearity of the assay method over time in the concentration area of the cutoff. After acceptable values are obtained for the known calibrators, those values will be used to calculate sample data. A minimum of 10% of the total specimens and quality control samples in each analytical run will be quality control samples. And 1% of each run, with a minimum of at least one sample, shall be the laboratory's blind quality control samples to appear as normal samples to the laboratory analysts. Implementation of procedures to ensure that carryover does not contaminate the testing of a donor's specimen shall be documented.

e. *Personnel:* The laboratory shall have a responsible person (ie, laboratory director) to assume professional, organizational, educational, and administrative responsibility for the laboratory's urine drug testing facility. This individual shall have documented scientific qualifications in analytical forensic toxicology. Minimum qualifications are certification as a laboratory director by the state in forensic or clinical laboratory toxicology; or a doctorate in one of the natural sciences with an adequate undergraduate and graduate education in biology, chemistry, and pharmacology or toxicology; or training and experience comparable to a doctorate in one of the natural sciences, such as a medical or scientific degree with additional training and laboratory/research experience in biology, chemistry, and pharmacology or toxicology. In addition to these requirements, minimum qualifications also require: appropriate experience in analytical forensic toxicology including experience with the analysis of biological material for drugs of abuse, and appropriate training and/or experience in forensic applications of analytical toxicology, such as publications, court testimony, research concerning analytical toxicology of drugs of abuse, or other factors that qualify the individual as an expert witness in forensic toxicology. This individual shall be engaged in and responsible for the day-to-day management of the drug testing laboratory (even where another individual has overall responsibility for an entire multispecialty laboratory); ensuring that there are enough personnel with adequate training and experience to supervise and conduct the work of the drug testing laboratory; the continued competency of laboratory personnel by documenting their inservice training, reviewing their work performance, and verifying their skills; the laboratory's procedure manual (complete, up-to-date, available for personnel performing tests, and followed by those personnel, reviewed, signed, and dated by the responsible person whenever procedures are first placed into use or changed or when a new individual assumes responsibility for management of the drug testing laboratory); maintaining a quality assurance program to ensure the proper performance and reporting of all test results; maintaining acceptable analytical performance for all controls and standards; maintaining quality control testing; ensuring and documenting the validity, reliability, accuracy, precision, and performance characteristics of each test and test system; taking all remedial actions necessary to maintain satisfactory operation and performance of the laboratory in response to quality control systems not being within performance specifications, errors in result reporting or in analysis of performance testing results; and ensuring that sample results are not reported until all corrective actions have been taken and he or she can ensure that the results provided are accurate and reliable. The laboratory's urine drug testing facility shall have a certifying scientist(s), who reviews all pertinent data and quality control results in order to attest to the validity of the laboratory's test reports. A laboratory may designate certifying scientists that are qualified to certify only results that are negative on the initial test and certifying scientists that are qualified to certify both initial and confirmatory tests. The laboratory's urine drug testing facility shall have an individual(s) to be responsible for day-to-day operations and to supervise the technical analysts. This individual(s) shall have at least a bachelor's degree in the chemical or biological sciences or medical technology or equivalent. He or she shall have training and experience in the theory and practice of the procedures used in the laboratory, resulting in his or her thorough understanding of quality control practices and procedures; the review, interpretation, and reporting of test results; maintenance of chain of custody; and proper remedial actions to be taken in response to test systems being out of control limits or detecting aberrant test or quality control results. Other technicians or nontechnical staff shall have the necessary training and skills for the tasks assigned. The laboratory's urine drug testing program shall make available continuing education programs to meet the needs of laboratory personnel. Laboratory personnel files shall include resume of training and experience; certification or license, if any; references; job descriptions; records of performance evaluation and advancement; incident reports; and results of tests that establish employee competency for the position he or she holds, such as a test for color blindness, if appropriate.

f. *Inspections:* The NLCP administers its own inspection program. To become certified initially, an applicant laboratory successfully complete a laboratory inspection that occurs at the time the third set of initial PT samples are being tested by the laboratory. In addition, the newly certified laboratory must undergo an inspection 3 months after achieving certification. To maintain certification, it must achieve successful performance on every subsequent semiannual "maintenance" inspection. The secretary of the DHHS, any federal agency utilizing the laboratory, or any organization performing laboratory certification on behalf of the secretary may reserve the right to inspect the laboratory at any time. Agency contracts with laboratories for drug testing, as well as contracts for collection site services, shall permit the agency to conduct unannounced inspections. In addition, prior to the award of a contract the agency may carry out preaward inspections and evaluation of the procedural aspects of the laboratory's drug testing operation.[36]

SUMMARY

In the United States, nationally recognized accreditation is a prerequisite for operating any toxicology laboratory performing testing on human specimens. The specific official form this accreditation takes and the pathway(s) to its achievement and maintenance differ between clinical and forensic toxicology laboratories, but in the broadest outline, analogous requirements exist in comparable areas of compliance for both types of operations.

REFERENCES

1. Department of Health and Human Services, Centers for Medicare & Medicaid Services. Part 493 Laboratory requirements, clinical laboratory improvement amendments of 1988, subpart A, sec. 493.1, basis and scope, 42CFR493.1, revised as of October 1, 2004.
2. Department of Health and Human Services, Centers for Medicare & Medicaid Services. Part 493 Laboratory requirements, clinical laboratory improvement amendments of 1988, subpart A, sec. 493.3(b) and (c), applicability, 42CFR493.3(b) and (c), revised as of October 1, 2004.
3. Department of Health and Human Services, Centers for Medicare & Medicaid Services. Part 493 Laboratory requirements, clinical laboratory improvement amendments of 1988, subpart A, sec. 493.2, definitions, 42CFR493.2, revised as of October 1, 2004.
4. Department of Health and Human Services, Centers for Medicare & Medicaid Services, Part 493 Laboratory requirements, clinical laboratory improvement amendments of 1988, subpart A, sec. 493.5(c), categories of test by complexity, 42CFR493.5(c), revised as of October 1, 2004.
5. Washington State Department of Health, Laboratory Quality Assurance. Available at: http://www.doh.wa.gov/LicensesPermitsandCertificates/FacilitiesNewRenewor Update/LaboratoryQualityAssurance.aspx. Accessed June 14, 2012.
6. New York State Department of Health, Wadsworth Center, Division of Laboratory Quality Certification. Clinical Laboratory Evaluation Program (CLEP). http://www.wadsworth.org/labcert/clep/clep.html. Accessed June 14, 2012.
7. Department of Health and Human Services, Centers for Medicare & Medicaid Services. Part 493 Laboratory requirements, clinical laboratory improvement amendments of 1988, subpart A, sec. 493.15 laboratories performing waived tests.
8. U.S. Food and Drug Administration. CLIA Currently Waived Analytes. Available at: http://www.accessdata.fda.gov/scripts/cdrh/cfdocs/cfClia/analyteswaived.cfm. Accessed June 14, 2012.
9. Department of Health and Human Services, Centers for Medicare & Medicaid Services. Part 493 Laboratory requirements, clinical laboratory improvement amendments of 1988, subpart H, participation in proficiency testing for laboratories performing nonwaived testing, sec. 493.801 through 493.865.

10. Accutest Inc., Wooster, MA. CLIA Approved Proficiency Testing Programs 2012. Available at: http://www.cms.hhs.gov/CLIA/downloads/ptlist.pdf. Accessed June 14, 2012.

11. Department of Health and Human Services, Centers for Medicare & Medicaid Services. Part 493 Laboratory requirements, clinical laboratory improvement amendments of 1988, subpart J, Sec. 493.1100 through 493.1105, facility administration for nonwaived testing, 42CFR493.1105, revised as of October 1, 2004.

12. Department of Health and Human Services, Occupational Safety and Health Administration. Air Contaminants – Permissible Exposure Limits, OSHA, 29 CFR 1910.1000.

13. Department of Health and Human Services, Occupational Safety and Health Administration. General Housekeeping requirements, OSHA, 29 CFR 1910.22.

14. Department of Health and Human Services, Occupational Safety and Health Administration. Hazard communication standard, OSHA, 29 CFR 1910.1200.

15. Department of Health and Human Services, Occupational Safety and Health Administration. Occupational exposure to bloodborne pathogens, needlesticks and other sharps injuries, final rule, January 18, 2001, 29 CFR 1910; occupational exposure to bloodborne pathogens, OSHA, 29 CFR 1910.1030.

16. Department of Health and Human Services, Occupational Safety and Health Administration. Occupational exposure to hazardous chemicals in laboratories, OSHA, 29 CFR 1910.1450.

17. Department of Health and Human Services, Occupational Safety and Health Administration. Occupational injury and illness recording and reporting requirement, 29 CFR 1904 and 29 CFR 1952.

18. Department of Health and Human Services, Occupational Safety and Health Administration. Personal protective equipment, OSHA, 29 CFR 1910.132.

19. Department of Health and Human Services, Occupational Safety and Health Administration. Sanitation, waste disposal, OSHA, 29 CFR 1910.141.

20. Department of Health and Human Services, Occupational Safety and Health Administration. Specifications for accident prevention signs and tags, OSHA, 29 CFR 1910.145.

21. Medical Waste Tracking Act of 1988. Standards for the tracking and management of medical waste, authority, 42 USC 69192,6992 et seq.

22. Health Insurance Portability and Accountability Act of 1996. 45 CFR Parts 160,162 and 164 as amended February 16, 2006.

23. Department of Health and Human Services, Centers for Medicare & Medicaid Services. Part 493 Laboratory requirements, clinical laboratory improvement amendments of 1988, subpart K, sec. 493.1105, standard: retention requirements, 42CFR493.1105, Revised as of October 1, 2004.

24. Department of Health and Human Services, Centers for Medicare & Medicaid Services. Part 493 Laboratory requirements, clinical laboratory improvement amendments of 1988, subpart K, sec. 493.1200, facility administration for nonwaived testing, 42CFR493.1200, revised as of October 1, 2004.

25. College of American Pathologists. Requirement FDT.00837, forensic drug testing checklist, revised June 15, 2009. Available at: http://www.cap.org/apps/docs/laboratory_accreditation/checklists/FDT_web_may2007.pdf. Accessed June 14, 2012.

26. Department of Health and Human Services, Centers for Medicare & Medicaid Services. Part 493 Laboratory requirements, clinical laboratory improvement amendments of 1988, subpart L, sec. 493.1445(e)(1) through sec. 493.1445(e15), laboratory director responsibilities, 42CFR493.1455(e).

27. Department of Health and Human Services, Centers for Medicare & Medicaid Services. Part 493 Laboratory requirements, clinical laboratory improvement amendments of 1988, subpart M, sec. 493.1451(b)(8) through (b)(9), facility administration for nonwaived testing, 42CFR493.1451, revised as of October 1, 2004.
28. College of American Pathologists. Accreditation and Laboratory Improvement. Available at: http://www.cap.org/apps/cap.portal?_nfpb=true&_pageLabel=accreditation. Accessed June 14, 2012.
29. American Board of Forensic Toxicology. Available at: http://www.abft.org. Accessed June 14, 2012.
30. American Society of Crime Laboratory Directors/Laboratory Accreditation Board. Available at: http://www.asclad-lab.net. Accessed June 14, 2012.
31. Department of Health and Human Services, Substance Abuse and Mental Health Services Administration, Center for Substance Abuse Prevention. National Laboratory Certification Program (NLCP). Available at: http://dwp.samsha.gov/DrugTesting/pdf/Natl_Lab_Cert_Prog_Background1007.pdf. Accessed June 14, 2012.
32. College of American Pathologists. Standards for Forensic Drug Testing Laboratory Accreditation. Available at: http://www.cap.org/apps/docs/laboratory_accreditation/forensic_urine.pdf. Accessed June 14, 2012.
33. American Board of Forensic Toxicology. Laboratory Accreditation. Available at: http://www.abft.org/index.php?option=com_content&view=article&id=51&Itemid=60. Accessed June 14, 2012.
34. Association of State Crime Lab Directors. Laboratory Accreditation Board. International Testing Forms. Available at: http://www.ascld-lab.org/forms/forms_intl.html. Accessed June 14, 2012.
35. International Organization for Standardization. ISO/IEC 17025:2005. Available at: http://www.iso.org/iso/catalogue_detail.htm?csnumber=39883. Accessed June 14, 2012.
36. Department of Health and Human Services, Substance Abuse and Mental Health Services Administration, Center for Substance Abuse Prevention. Mandatory guidelines for federal workplace drug testing programs (mandatory guidelines). 53 CFR 11970 April 11, 1988; subsequently revised June 9, 1994 (59 CFR 29908); September 30, 1997 (62 CFR 51118); April 13, 2004 (69 CFR 19644); November 25, 2008 (73 CFR 71858); December 10, 2008 (73 CFR 75122); and on April 30, 2010 (75 CFR 22809).

Index

Note: Page numbers of article titles are in **boldface** type.

A

Accreditation, for toxicology testing, **525–542**
  clinical laboratory, 526–532
    CLIA certification, 526
    CLIA-exempt, 526–527
    inspection in, 532
    nonwaived testing in, 527–532
    personnel for, 530–532
    proficiency testing in, 527–530
    waived testing in, 527
  forensic, 494–495, 532–540
    American Board of Forensic Toxicology Laboratory Accreditation Program (ABFT) for, 534–536
    American Society of Crime Laboratory Directors Laboratory Accreditation Board (ASCLD/LAB) program for, 536–537
    CAP program for, 533–534
    legal implications of, 533
    Substance Abuse and Mental Health Services Administration (SAMHSA) National Laboratory Certification Program for, 537–540
Accuracy, of method, in forensic toxicology, 498–499
6-Acetylmorphine, immunoassay screen for, 440
ADRB2 gene polymorphisms, 511
Alanine aminotransferase, as alcohol biomarker, 394–396
Alcohol use disorders, **391–406**
  acute effects of, 392
  biomarkers for
    alternate specimen types for, 400–402
    direct, 396–400
    indirect, 394–396
  chronic effects of, 392
  dependence in, 392–393
  epidemiology of, 392
  ethanol metabolism and, 393
  hair testing for, 479, 481
  neonatal exposure to, 461–462
  oral fluid testing in, 472–474
  pharmacogenomics in, 517
  physiologic effects of, 392–393
  teratogenic effects of, 393
  tolerance in, 392–393
Aldehyde adducts, as alcohol biomarkers, 396–397
Alprazolam, abuse of, 367–371

Clin Lab Med 32 (2012) 543–555
http://dx.doi.org/10.1016/S0272-2712(12)00102-3
0272-2712/12/$ – see front matter © 2012 Elsevier Inc. All rights reserved.
labmed.theclinics.com